BRAIN MAKER

BRAIN MAKER

The Power of Gut Microbes to Heal and

Protect Your Brain — for Life

BY DAVID PERLMUTTER, MD

WITH KRISTIN LOBERG

LITTLE, BROWN AND COMPANY

NEW YORK BOSTON LONDON

Copyright © 2015 by David Perlmutter, MD

All rights reserved. In accordance with the U.S. Copyright Act of 1976, the scanning, uploading, and electronic sharing of any part of this book without the permission of the publisher constitute unlawful piracy and theft of the author's intellectual property. If you would like to use material from the book (other than for review purposes), prior written permission must be obtained by contacting the publisher at permissions@hbgusa.com. Thank you for your support of the author's rights.

Little, Brown and Company
Hachette Book Group
1290 Avenue of the Americas, New York, NY 10104
littlebrown.com

First Edition: April 2015

Little, Brown and Company is a division of Hachette Book Group, Inc. The Little, Brown name and logo are trademarks of Hachette Book Group, Inc.

The publisher is not responsible for websites (or their content) that are not owned by the publisher.

The Hachette Speakers Bureau provides a wide range of authors for speaking events. To find out more, go to hachettespeakersbureau.com or call (866) 376-6591.

ISBN 978-0-316-38010-2
Library of Congress Control Number 2015933527

RRD-H

Printed in the United States of America

10 9 8 7 6 5 4 3 2 1

This book is dedicated to you. Just as the multitude of organisms
residing within your body sustains you, so too does each
and every individual influence the well-being of our planet. In a very
real sense, you are an active member of the earth's microbiome.

"No man is an island,
entire of itself . . ."
— JOHN DONNE

Contents

PART I

GETTING TO KNOW YOUR HUNDRED TRILLION FRIENDS

Contents

BRAIN MAKER

Bug Alert: You've Got Company

Death begins in the colon.
— ÉLIE MECHNIKOV (1845–1916)

SEVERAL TIMES A WEEK THROUGHOUT my career, I've had to tell a patient or caregiver that there's nothing left in my arsenal to treat a grave neurological disease that will inevitably shatter the patient's life. I've surrendered because the illness gained too much control and no quick fix or drug existed to even decelerate the swift march of the affliction to the end. It's a heart-wrenching place to be, one that you just don't get used to no matter how many times you go through it. What gives me hope, however, is a burgeoning area of study that's finally affording me revolutionary approaches to relieving the suffering. *Brain Maker* is about this dazzling new science, and how you can take advantage of it for your own health.

Take a moment to think about how much has changed in our world over the past century, thanks to medical research. No longer do we worry about dying from smallpox, dysentery, diphtheria, cholera, or scarlet fever. We've made huge strides in lowering the death rates of many life-threatening maladies, including HIV/AIDS, some forms of cancer, and heart disease. But when you consider brain-related diseases and disorders, the picture is vastly different. Advances in preventing, treating, and curing debilitating neurological ailments across the life cycle — from autism and attention deficit hyperactivity disorder (ADHD) to migraines, depression, multiple sclerosis (MS), Parkinson's, and Alzheimer's — are virtually nonexistent. And, sadly, we are quickly losing ground as the incidences of these conditions are increasing in our society.

Let's consider a few numbers. In the ten wealthiest Western nations, death from brain disease in general, which largely reflects death from dementia, has risen dramatically over the past twenty years. And the United States leads the way. In fact, a 2013 British report showed that since 1979, death due to brain disease increased a breathtaking 66 percent in men and 92 percent in women in America. In the words of the study's lead author, Professor Colin Prichard, "These statistics are about real people and families, and we need to [recognize] that there is an 'epidemic' that clearly is influenced by environmental and societal changes." The researchers also noted how this surge, which is affecting people at younger and younger ages, is in sharp contrast to the major reductions in risk of death from all other causes.[1]

In 2013, the *New England Journal of Medicine* published a report revealing that we spend about $50,000 annually caring for each dementia patient in this country.[2] That amounts to approximately $200 billion a year, twice what we spend on caring for heart disease patients and almost triple what we spend on treatment for cancer patients.

Mood and anxiety disorders are also on the upswing and can be equally as crippling to quality of life as other neurological conditions. About one in four adults in the U.S. — more than 26 percent of the population — suffers from a diagnosable mental disorder.[3] Anxiety disorders afflict more than 40 million Americans, and nearly 10 percent of the U.S. adult population has a mood disorder for which powerful drugs are prescribed.[4] Depression, which affects one in ten of us (including a quarter of women in their forties and fifties), is now the leading cause of disability worldwide, and diagnoses are growing at a startling rate.[5]

4

Medications like Prozac and Zoloft are among the most often prescribed drugs in the nation. Mind you, these drugs treat *symptoms* of depression, not the causes, which are flagrantly ignored. On average, people with severe mental illness, such as bipolar disorder and schizophrenia, die twenty-five years earlier than the general population.[6] (This is partially due to the fact that these individuals are more likely to smoke, abuse alcohol and drugs, and be overweight with obesity-related illnesses in addition to their mental challenges.)

Headaches, including migraines, are among the most common disorders of the nervous system; nearly half of the adult population wrestles with at least one headache per month. And they are more than an inconvenience; they are associated with disability, personal suffering, damaged quality of life, and financial cost.[7] We tend to think of headaches as being inexpensive nuisances, especially since many drugs that treat them are relatively cheap and easy to access (e.g., aspirin, acetaminophen, ibuprofen), but according to the National Pain Foundation, they cause more than 160 million lost work days each year in the U.S. and result in about $30 billion a year in medical expenses.[8]

Multiple sclerosis, a disabling autoimmune disease that disrupts the nervous system's ability to communicate, now affects an estimated two and a half million people worldwide, with close to half a million in America, and is becoming increasingly more prevalent.[9] The average lifetime cost of treating someone with MS exceeds $1.2 million.[10] Mainstream medicine tells us that there is no cure in sight.

And then there is autism, which has surged seven- to eight-fold just in the past 15 years, making this truly a modern-day epidemic.[11]

To be sure, hundreds of millions of dollars are being spent on these and other enfeebling brain-related ailments, yet we are seeing precious little progress.

Now for the good news: New, leading-edge science coming from the most well-respected institutions around the world is discovering that to an extraordinary degree, brain health and, on the flip side, brain diseases, are dictated by what goes on in the gut. That's right: what's taking place in your intestines today is determining your risk for any number of neurological conditions. I realize this may be difficult to comprehend; if you were to ask your doctors about a known cure for autism, MS, depression, or dementia, they would throw up their arms and say none exists—and may never exist.

It is here that I part company with most, but gratefully not all, of my colleagues. We as neurologists are trained to focus on what goes on in the nervous system, and specifically in the brain, in a myopic way. We automatically end up viewing other bodily systems, such as the gastrointestinal tract, as discrete entities that have no bearing whatsoever on what goes on in the brain. After all, when you have a stomachache you don't call a cardiologist or neurologist. The entire medical industry is characterized by distinct disciplines divided by body part or individual system. Most of my colleagues would say, "What happens in the gut stays in the gut."

This perspective is grossly out of touch with current science. The digestive system is intimately connected to what goes on in the brain. And perhaps the most important aspect of the gut that has *everything* to do with your general wellness and mental health is its internal ecology—the various microorganisms that live within it, especially the bacteria.

MEET YOUR MICROBIOME

Historically, we've been taught to think of bacteria as agents of death. The bubonic plague, after all, wiped out nearly one third of the population in Europe between 1347 and 1352, and certain bacterial infections are still worldwide killers today. But the time has come to embrace another side of bacteria's story in our lives. We must consider how some bugs are not detrimental but fundamental to life.

The Greek physician and father of modern medicine, Hippocrates, first said in the third century B.C.E., "All disease begins in the gut." This was long before civilization had any proof or sound theory to explain this idea. We didn't even know bacteria existed until the Dutch tradesman and scientist Antonie van Leeuwenhoek looked at his own dental plaque through a handcrafted microscope in the late 17th century and spied a hidden world of what he called "animalcules." Today he is considered the father of microbiology.

In the nineteenth century it was the Russian-born biologist and Nobel laureate Élie Mechnikov who made a stunningly direct link between human longevity and a healthy balance of bacteria in the body, confirming that "death begins in the colon." Since his discoveries, made at a time when bloodletting was still popular, scientific research is bringing more and more credence to the notion that up to 90 percent of all known human illness can be traced back to an unhealthy gut. And we can say for sure that just as disease begins in the gut, so too does health and vitality. It was also Mechnikov who said that the good bacteria must outnumber the bad. Unfortunately, most people today carry around more bad, pathogenic bacteria than they should, lacking an abundant and diverse microbial universe within. No wonder we suffer from so many brain disorders.

If only Mechnikov were alive today to be a part of the next medical revolution that he tried to start in the nineteenth century. This one is finally under way.

Right now, your body is colonized by a multitude of organisms that outnumber your own cells by a factor of about ten (luckily, our cells are much larger, so those organisms don't outweigh us ten to one!). These roughly hundred trillion invisible creatures—microbes—cover your insides and outsides, thriving in your mouth, nose, ears, intestines, genitalia, and on every inch of your skin. If you could isolate them all, they would fill up a half-gallon container. Scientists have so far identified some 10,000 species of microbes, and because each microbe contains its own DNA, that translates to more than eight million genes. In other words, for every human gene in your body, there are at least 360 microbial ones.[12]

Most of these organisms live within your digestive tract, and while they include fungi and viruses, it appears that the bacterial species that make their home inside you dominate and take center stage in supporting every conceivable aspect of your health. And you interact not only with these organisms but also with their genetic material.

We call this complex internal ecology that thrives within us and its genetic fingerprint the microbiome (*micro* for "small" or "microscopic," *biome* referring to a naturally occurring community of flora occupying a large habitat—in this case, the human body). Although the human genome we all carry is almost the same, give or take the small handful of genes that encode our individual characteristics like hair color or blood type, the gut microbiome of even identical twins is vastly different. Research at the leading edge of medicine is now acknowledging that the state of the microbiome is so key to human health—with a sweeping say in whether or not you live robustly to a ripe old age—that it should be considered an organ in and of itself. And it's an organ that has gone through radical changes over the past two-plus million years. We have evolved to have an intimate, symbiotic relationship with these microbial inhabitants who have actively participated in shaping our evolution since the dawn of humankind (and indeed, they lived on the planet for billions of years prior to our emergence). At the same time, they have adapted and changed in response to the environments we have created for them within our bodies. Even the expression of our genes in each and every one of our cells is influenced to some degree by these bacteria and other organisms that live within us.

The importance of the microbiome motivated the National Institutes of Health (NIH) to launch the Human Microbiome Project in 2008 as an extension of the Human Genome Project.[13] Some of America's best scientists have been charged with exploring how changes in the microbiome are associated with health and, conversely, disease. Moreover, they are studying what can be done with this information to help reverse many of our most challenging health problems. Although the project is investigating several parts of the body that host microbes, including the skin, the most extensive area of research is focused on the gut since it's home to most of your body's microbes and, as you're about to discover, a center of gravity of sorts for your entire physiology.

It's now undeniable that our intestinal organisms participate in a wide variety of physiologic actions, including immune system functioning, detoxification, inflammation, neurotransmitter and vitamin production, nutrient absorption, signaling being hungry or full, and utilizing carbohydrates and fat. All of these processes factor mightily into whether or not we experience allergies, asthma, ADHD, cancer, diabetes, or dementia. The microbiome affects our mood, libido, metabolism, immunity, and even our perception of the world and the clarity of our thoughts. It helps determine whether we are fat or thin, energetic or lethargic. Put simply, everything about our health—how we feel both emotionally and physically—hinges on the state of our microbiome. Is it healthy and dominated by so-called friendly, beneficial bacteria? Or is it sick and overrun by bad, unfriendly bacteria?

Perhaps no other system in the body is more sensitive to changes in gut bacteria than the central nervous system, especially the brain. In 2014, the U.S. National Institute of Mental Health spent more than $1 million on a new research program zeroing in on the microbiome-brain connection.[14] Although many things factor into the health of our microbiome and therefore the health of our brain, nurturing a healthy microbiome today is easier than you think. I've taken all the guesswork out with the recommendations presented in this book.

I've seen dramatic turnarounds in health using simple dietary modifications and, on occasion, more aggressive techniques to reestablish a healthy microbiome. Take, for instance, the gentleman with such a horrid case of multiple sclerosis that he required a wheelchair and bladder catheter. After treatment, not only did he say goodbye to his catheter and regain the ability to walk without assistance, but his MS went into total remission. Or consider Jason, the 12-year-old boy with severe autism who could barely talk in full sentences. In chapter 5 you'll read about how he physically transformed into an engaging boy after a vigorous probiotic protocol. And I can't wait to share with you the countless stories of individuals with myriad, enfeebling health challenges—from chronic pain, fatigue, and depression to serious bowel disorders and autoimmune diseases—who experienced a complete vanishing of symptoms following treatment. They went from having an awful quality of life to getting a second chance. Some even went from harboring thoughts of suicide to feeling content and vivacious for the first time. These stories are not outlier cases for me, but by standard measure of what might typically be expected, they seem almost miraculous. I witness these stories every day, and I know that you too can positively change the fate of your brain through the health of your gut. In this book, I'll show you how.

Although you may not have extreme and unrelenting health challenges that require pharmaceuticals or intensive therapy, a dysfunctional microbiome could be at the root of your bothersome headaches, anxiety, inability to concentrate, or negative outlook on life. Drawing on scholarly clinical and laboratory studies, as well as extraordinary results I've seen over and over again or heard about at medical conferences that attract the finest physicians and scientists from around the world, I'll tell you what we know and how we can take advantage of this knowledge. I'll also offer highly practical and comprehensive guidelines to transform your gut health and in turn your cognitive health so you can add many more vibrant years to your life. And the benefits don't stop there. This new science can help all of the following:

- ADHD
- Asthma
- Autism
- Allergies and food sensitivities
- Chronic fatigue

- Mood disorders, including depression and anxiety

- Diabetes and cravings for sugar and carbohydrates

- Overweight and obesity, as well as weight-loss struggles

- Memory problems and poor concentration

- Chronic constipation or diarrhea

- Frequent colds or infections

- Intestinal disorders, including celiac disease, irritable bowel syndrome, and Crohn's disease

- Insomnia

- Painful joint inflammations and arthritis

- High blood pressure

- Atherosclerosis

- Chronic yeast problems

- Skin problems such as acne and eczema

- Bad breath, gum disease, and dental problems

- Tourette syndrome

- Extreme menstrual and menopausal symptoms

- And many more

In fact, this new knowledge can help virtually any degenerative or inflammatory condition.

In the pages that follow we will explore what makes for a healthy microbiome and what makes a good microbiome go bad. The quiz on page 16 will clue you into the kinds of lifestyle factors and circumstances that relate directly to the health and function of the microbiome. And one thing you'll grasp quickly is that food really does matter.

YOU ARE WHAT YOU EAT

The idea that food is the most important variable in human health is not news. As the old adage goes, "Let food be thy medicine and medicine be thy food."[15] Anyone can change the state of their microbiome—and fate of their health—through dietary choices.

I recently had the opportunity to interview Dr. Alessio Fasano, who currently serves as visiting professor at Harvard Medical School and Chief of the Division of Pediatric Gastroenterology and Nutrition at Massachusetts General Hospital. He is recognized as a global thought leader in the science of the microbiome. We spoke about factors that alter gut bacteria, and he stated clearly to me that, hands down, the most significant factor related to the health and diversity of the microbiome is the food we eat. And what we put in our mouths represents the biggest environmental challenge to our genome and the microbiome.

What a massive endorsement for the notion that food matters, trumping other circumstances in our life that we may not entirely be able to control.

As I described in my previous book *Grain Brain*, the two key mechanisms that lead to brain degeneration are chronic inflammation and the action of free radicals, which for now you can think of as byproducts of inflammation that cause the body to "rust." *Brain Maker* takes a new look at these mechanisms and how they are influenced by gut bacteria and your overall gut health. Your intestinal flora in fact has everything to do with inflammation and whether or not you can combat free radicals. In other words, the state of your microbiome determines whether or not your body is fanning the flames of inflammation or squelching them.

Chronic inflammation and free radical damage are concepts that lie front and center in neuroscience today, but no pharmaceutical approach can come anywhere close to a dietary prescription for managing your intestinal bacteria. I'll explain that prescription step by step. Thankfully, the gut's microbiotic community is wonderfully receptive to rehabilitation.

The guidelines outlined in this book will change your body's inner ecology to enhance the growth of the right kind of brain-sustaining organisms. This highly practical regimen includes six essential keys: prebiotics, probiotics, fermented foods, low-carb foods, gluten-free foods, and healthful fat. I'll explain how each of these factors plays into the health of the microbiome for the benefit of the brain.

Best of all, you can reap the rewards of the *Brain Maker* protocol within a matter of weeks.

GET READY

I have absolutely no doubt in my mind that by embracing this information, we will completely revolutionize the treatment of neurological illnesses. And I can't express in words how honored I feel to be able to present these revelations to the public, exposing all the data that's been quietly circulating in the medical literature. You're about to appreciate how your microbiome is the ultimate brain maker.

My recommendations in this book are designed to treat and prevent brain disorders; alleviate moodiness, anxiety, and depression; bolster your immune system and reduce autoimmunity; and improve metabolic disorders, including diabetes and obesity, which factor into long-term brain health. I'm going to describe aspects of your life that you might never have guessed take part in your brain health. I'll discuss the significance of your birth story, of your nutrition and prescribed medications as a child, and of your hygiene habits (for example, your use of hand sanitizers). I'll explore how gut bacteria are different in populations around the world and how these differences are caused by dissimilarities in diet. I'll even take you through what our ancestors ate thousands of years ago and how this relates to new research about the microbiome. We will consider the notion of urbanization: how has it changed our internal ecological community? Has sanitized city living led to increased rates of autoimmune disease? I trust that you'll find this discussion equally illuminating and empowering.

I will show you how food-borne prebiotics—nutrient sources of fuel for the beneficial bacteria that live within your gut—play fundamental roles in preserving health by maintaining balance and diversity of intestinal bacteria. Foods such as garlic, Jerusalem artichoke, jicama, and even dandelion greens, as well as fermented foods such as sauerkraut, kombucha, and kimchi open the door for heightened levels of health in general, and brain function and protection in particular.

Although probiotics have now become commonplace in many food products and can be found in regular grocery stores, it helps to know how to navigate all the options—especially when you're confronted with "good for the gut" advertising. I'll help you do just that, explaining the science behind probiotics and how to choose the best ones.

Of course, other lifestyle habits factor into the equation, too. In addition to exploring the interaction between the microbiome and brain, we'll be getting to know a new discipline: epigenetic medicine. This science examines how lifestyle choices such as diet, exercise, sleep, and stress management influence the expression of our DNA and play directly and indirectly into brain health. I will also share with you the role of mitochondria in brain disorders, from the perspective of the microbiome. The mitochondria are tiny structures within our cells that have their own DNA separate from the DNA in the nuclei. The mitochondria can in fact be considered a third dimension to our microbiome; they have a unique relationship with the microbiome in our guts.

Parts 1 and 2 will provide the foundation you need to embark on my brain maker rehab program in part 3. I've given you a lot of information in this introduction. I hope I've begun to whet your appetite for learning about and embracing this whole new area of medicine, a fresh approach to maintaining brain health. Nothing but a stronger, brighter, healthier future awaits you.

Let's get started.

What Are Your Risk Factors?

WHILE THERE'S NO SINGLE TEST available today that can accurately tell you the state of your microbiome, you can gather clues by answering a few simple questions. These questions can also help you understand which experiences in your life—from your birth to today—may have impacted the health of your gut.

Note: Although microbial testing kits are starting to emerge on the market, I don't think the research is there yet in terms of knowing what the results truly mean (healthy vs. unhealthy) and which risk factors you bear. In the future I have no doubt we'll be able to establish evidence-based parameters and defined correlations between certain microbial signatures and conditions. But for now this is tricky terrain; it's still too early to know whether certain patterns being studied in the gut microbiome that are related to illness X or disorder Y are part of the cause or the effect of those conditions. That said, these kits can be useful for gauging the diversity and general composition of your microbiome. But even then, it can be difficult to say that a certain microbial makeup identifies you as "healthy." And I wouldn't want you to try to understand the results from such tests on your own without proper guidance from trained medical professionals who are experienced in this domain. So for now, I'd press pause until further notice about these kits. The questions below will arm you with plenty of personal data that can help provide a sense of your risk factors.

Don't be alarmed if you find yourself answering yes to most of these questions. The more yeses you have, the higher your risk might be for having a sick or dysfunctional microbiome that could be impacting your mental health, but you are not doomed. My whole point in writing this book is to empower you to take charge of your gut's health and, in turn, your brain's health.

If you don't know the answer to a question, skip over it. And if any particular one alarms you or prompts you to ask further questions, rest assured I will answer them in the upcoming chapters. For now, just respond to these questions to the best of your ability.

1. Did your mother take antibiotics while she was pregnant with you?

2. Did your mother take steroids like prednisone while she was pregnant with you?

3. Were you born by C-section?

4. Were you breast-fed for less than one month?

5. Did you suffer from frequent ear and/or throat infections as a child?

6. Did you require ear tubes as a child?

7. Did you have your tonsils removed?

8. Have you ever needed steroid medications for more than one week, including steroid nasal or breathing inhalers?

9. Do you take antibiotics at least once every two to three years?

10. Do you take acid-blocking drugs (for digestion or reflux)?

11. Are you gluten-sensitive?

12. Do you have food allergies?

13. Are you extra sensitive to chemicals often found in everyday products and goods?

14. Have you been diagnosed with an autoimmune disease?

15. Do you have type-2 diabetes?

16. Are you more than 20 pounds overweight?

17. Do you suffer from irritable bowel syndrome?

18. Do you have diarrhea or loose bowel movements at least once a month?

19. Do you require a laxative at least once a month?

20. Do you suffer from depression?

I bet you're curious now as to what all this means. This book will tell you everything you want — and need — to know, and so much more.

PART I

GETTING TO KNOW YOUR HUNDRED TRILLION FRIENDS

THEY DON'T HAVE EYES, EARS, noses, or teeth. They don't have limbs, hearts, livers, lungs, or brains. They don't breathe or eat like we do. You can't even see them with the naked eye. But don't underestimate them. On the one hand, bacteria are amazingly simple, each consisting of only a single cell. On the other hand, they are extraordinarily complex, even sophisticated in many ways, and they are a fascinating group of creatures. Don't let their infinitesimally small size fool you. Some bacteria can live in temperatures that would boil your blood, and others thrive in below-freezing places. One species can even tolerate radiation levels thousands of times greater than you could withstand. These microscopic living cells feast on everything from sugar and starch to sunlight and sulfur. Bacteria are the foundation of all life on earth. They were the planet's original life forms, and they will probably be the last. Why? Absolutely nothing living can exist without them, not even you.

While you're probably familiar with the fact that certain bacteria can cause disease and even kill, you might not be so attuned to the other side of the story—that our every heartbeat, exhalation, and neuronal connection helps bacteria sustain human life. Not only do these bacteria coexist with us—coating our insides and outsides—but they help our bodies perform a breathtaking array of functions necessary to our survival.

In part I, we're going to explore the human microbiome—what it is, how it works, and the incredible relationship between your gut's microbial community and your brain. You'll learn how conditions as diverse as autism, depression, dementia, and even cancer share a lot in common, thanks to gut bacteria. We'll also look at the factors key to the development of a healthy microbiome, as well as those that can compromise it. You'll soon begin to see that we likely owe our modern plagues, from obesity to Alzheimer's disease, to our sick and dysfunctional microbiome. By the end of this part, you'll have a new appreciation for your gut bacteria and a renewed sense of empowerment for the future of your health.

CHAPTER 1

Welcome Aboard

Your Microbial Friends from Birth to Death

SOMEWHERE ON A BEAUTIFUL GREEK island in the Aegean Sea, a baby boy is born at home naturally. He is breast-fed for two years. Growing up, he doesn't have many of the modern conveniences of American culture. Fast food, fruit juice, and soda are highly unusual fare for him. His meals consist mainly of vegetables from his family's garden, local fish and meat, homemade yogurt, nuts and seeds, and plenty of olive oil. He spends his childhood days learning in a small school and helping his parents on their farm, where they grow greens, herbs for making tea, and grapes for wine. The air is clean and there's no pollution.

When he gets sick, his parents give him a spoonful of locally produced honey, for antibiotics are not always available. He will never be diagnosed with autism, asthma, or attention deficit hyperactivity disorder. He stays fit and lean since it is common practice to be active. Families don't sit on couches at night; they often socialize with neighbors and dance to music. This boy will probably never be faced with a serious brain disorder such as depression or Alzheimer's disease. In fact, he will likely live to a ripe old age, as his island, Ikaria, is home to the highest percentage of ninety-year-olds on the planet—nearly one out of three people make it to their tenth decade in robust physical and mental health.[1] They also boast about 20 percent fewer cases of cancer, half the rate of heart disease, and almost no dementia.

Now let's go to any city in the U.S., where a baby girl is born. She enters the world via an elective C-section and is exclusively formula-fed. She endures multiple infections as a child—from chronic ear infections to throat and sinus infections—for which antibiotics are prescribed; she is prescribed antibiotics even for the common cold. Although she has access to the best nutrition in the world, her diet is overrun by processed foods, refined sugars, and unhealthy vegetable fats. By the time she's six years old, she is overweight and diagnosed as pre-diabetic. She matures into a savvy user of electronics and spends the majority of her youth at a rigorous school. But now she takes anti-anxiety medication, suffers from behavioral problems, and increasingly struggles with her academics because of her inability to focus. As an adult, she'll be at a high risk for grave brain-related conditions, including mood and anxiety disorders, migraines, and autoimmune disorders such as multiple sclerosis. And when she's older, she could face Parkinson's or Alzheimer's disease. In the U.S., the leading killers are related to chronic illnesses, such as dementia, rarely seen on that Greek island.

What's going on here? Over the past few years, new research has given us a much deeper understanding of the relationship between what we're exposed to from a very early age and our short- and long-term health. Scientists have been scrutinizing the links between the state of the human microbiome and the fate of one's health. The answer to the question lies in the difference between these two children's early life experience, and part of that experience, broadly speaking, has every-thing to do with the development of their individual microbiomes, the microbial communities that inhabit their bodies from birth and have a commanding role in health and brain function throughout life.

Obviously, I've taken some liberties in this hypothetical scenario.

There are a constellation of factors that figure into any single person's longevity and lifetime risk for certain diseases. But let's focus for a moment solely on the fact that the girl's early life experiences set her on an entirely different path in terms of brain health than the boy's. And yes, the Greek island really does exist. Ikaria lies about thirty miles off the western coast of Turkey. It's also known as a Blue Zone, a place where people live measurably longer, healthier lives than most of us in the Western developed world. They generally drink wine and coffee daily, stay active long past eighty years old, and remain mentally sharp to the very end. One prominent study found that Ikarian men are nearly four times as likely as their American counterparts to reach ninety, often in better health.[2] The study also found that they live up to a decade longer before developing cardiovascular disease and cancers, and they don't experience nearly as much depression. The rates of dementia in those past eighty-five years old are a small fraction of rates of Americans in this same age group.

I have no doubt that when science settles the score between these two vastly different places and we can tease out the root causes of our health challenges here in the U.S., the human microbiome will be at the forefront. I'll prove to you that it's as vital to your well-being as oxygen and water. What do your belly's bugs have to do with the brain and related diseases?

More than you ever imagined.

WHO'S IN CHARGE? YOUR GUT'S BUGS

Perhaps there's no better word for the microorganisms that live in your intestines and help with digestion than *superheroes*. Although it has been estimated that at least 10,000 distinct species cohabit the human gut, some experts argue that this number may exceed 35,000.[3] New technologies are finally emerging to help scientists identify all the species, many of which cannot be cultured in a laboratory via traditional methods.

For the purposes of this discussion, we're going to focus specifically on bacteria; they make up the majority of your gut microbes, alongside yeasts, viruses, protozoans, and eukaryotic parasites that also serve important, healthful roles. By and large, it's the bacteria that are your body's key players in collaborating with your physiology — especially your neurology. Collected together, the bacteria in your gut would weigh about three to four pounds, about the same weight as your brain (fully half of your stool weight is made up of discarded bacteria).[4]

When you think back to high school when you were studying the digestive system, you learned how it broke down foods into nutrients to be absorbed. You read about stomach acids and enzymes, as well as hormones that help guide the process. You probably had to memorize the steps that a typical morsel takes from the mouth to the anus. You may have even gotten as far as understanding how glucose — the sugar molecule — enters cells for use as energy. But you probably never heard about this veritable ecosystem living inside your digestive tract that pretty much commands the whole bodily system. You weren't tested on the gut bacteria whose DNA may have a much greater impact on your health than your own DNA.

I know, it's almost unbelievable. It sounds crazy, like science fiction. But the research is clear: Your gut's bugs may as well be considered an organ in their own right. And they are just as vital to your health as your own heart, lungs, liver, and brain. The latest science tells us that the intestinal flora that take up residence on the delicate folds of your intestinal walls

- Aid in digestion and the absorption of nutrients.

- Create a physical barrier against potential invaders such as bad bacteria (pathogenic flora), harmful viruses, and injurious parasites. Some types of bacteria have hair-like threads that help them swim; the "flagella," as these threads are called, have recently been shown to stop a deadly stomach rotavirus in its tracks.[5]

- Act as a detoxification machine. The gut's bugs have a role in preventing infections and serving as a line of defense against many toxins that make it down into your intestines. In fact, because they neutralize many toxins found in your food, they can be viewed as a second liver. So when you decrease the good bacteria in your gut, you increase the workload of your liver.

- Profoundly influence the immune system's response. Contrary to what you might think, the gut *is* your biggest immune system organ. Moreover, bacteria can educate and support the immune system by controlling certain immune cells and preventing autoimmunity (a state in which the body attacks its own tissues).

- Produce and release important enzymes and substances that collaborate with your biology, as well as chemicals for the brain, including vitamins and neurotransmitters.

- Help you handle stress through the flora's effects on your endocrine — hormonal — system.

- Assist you in getting a good night's sleep.

- Help control the body's inflammatory pathways, which in turn affect risk for virtually all manner of chronic disease.

Clearly, the good bacteria in a healthy gut are not squatters enjoying free food and lodging. They factor into risk not just for brain disorders and mental illness but also for cancer, asthma, food allergies, metabolic conditions such as diabetes and obesity, and autoimmune disease due to their direct and indirect influence on various organs and systems. Put simply, they are in charge of your health.

Some bacteria are more or less permanent residents; they form long-lasting colonies. Others are transient; but even the ones just passing through have important effects. Transient bacteria travel through the human digestive tract and, depending upon their type and unique characteristics, they have their say in the overall health of the body. But rather than take up permanent residence, they establish small colonies for brief periods of time before being excreted or dying off. In their temporary residence, however, they perform a large number of needed tasks; some of the substances they produce are critical to the health and wellness of the residential bacteria—and, in turn, of us.

THE ULTIMATE BRAIN MAKER

Although having a full understanding of the gut-brain connection demands a working knowledge of immunology, pathology, neurology, and endocrinology, I'm going to simplify it for you here. You will continue to build and reinforce this knowledge base as you read upcoming chapters.

Think of the last time you felt sick to your stomach because you were nervous, anxious, scared, or perhaps over-the-moon elated. Maybe it was before taking an important test, speaking before a group of people, or getting married. Scientists are just learning that the intimate relationship between your gut and brain is actually bidirectional: Just as your brain can send butterflies to your stomach, your gut can relay its state of calm or alarm to the nervous system.

The vagus nerve, the longest of the twelve cranial nerves, is the primary channel of information between the hundreds of millions of nerve cells in our intestinal nervous system and our central nervous system. Also known as cranial nerve X, it extends from the brain stem to the abdomen, directing many bodily processes that we don't consciously control. These include such important tasks as maintaining the heart rate and controlling digestion. And it turns out that the population of bacteria in the gut directly affects the stimulation and function of the cells along the vagus nerve. Some of the gut's microbes can actually release chemical messengers, just as our neurons do, that speak to the brain in their own language through the vagus nerve.

When you think of your nervous system, you probably picture your brain and spinal cord. But that's just the central nervous system. You must also consider your intestinal or enteric nervous system, the one that's intrinsic to the gastrointestinal tract. The central and enteric nervous systems are created from the same tissue during fetal development, and they are connected via the vagus nerve. *Vagus* means "wanderer," an apt name for this nerve, which wanders through the digestive system. (The word *vagabond* comes from the same root.)

The neurons in the gut are so innumerable that many scientists are now calling the totality of them "the second brain." Not only is this second brain regulating muscles, immune cells, and hormones, but it's also manufacturing something really important. Popular antidepressants like Paxil, Zoloft, and Lexapro increase the availability of the "feel-good" chemical serotonin in the brain. You may be surprised to find out that an estimated 80 to 90 percent of the amount of serotonin in your body is manufactured by the nerve cells in your gut![6] In fact, your gut's brain makes more serotonin—the master happiness molecule—than the brain in your head does. Many neurologists and psychiatrists are now realizing that this may be one reason why antidepressants are often less effective in treating depression than dietary changes are. In fact, recent research is revealing that our second brain may not be "second" at all.[7] It can act independently from the main brain and control many functions without the brain's input or help.

I'll explain more about the gut-brain's biology throughout the book. You'll learn about many biological functions in the upcoming chapters that all involve the microbiome. While some may seem wildly different from others, for example, what your immune cells are doing and how much insulin your pancreas is pumping out, you'll soon understand that they have the same common denominator: the gut's inhabitants. In many ways, they are your body's gatekeepers and rulers. They form your body's headquarters. They are the unsung heroes and partners in your health. And they are orchestrators of your physiology in ways you probably never imagined.

In connecting the dots from the gut to the brain, it helps to consider the body's general response to stress, both physical (e.g., running from an armed intruder in your house) and mental (e.g., avoiding an argument with your boss). Unfortunately, the body isn't clever enough to distinguish between the two, which is why your heart can pound just as hard before you prepare to run away from a burglar as when you're walking into your boss's office. Both scenarios are perceived as stress on the body, even though only one — escaping the intruder — is a real threat to survival. So in both instances your body will flood with natural steroids and adrenaline, and your immune system will release chemical messengers called inflammatory cytokines that send the system into high alert. This works well for episodic moments of duress, but what happens when the body is constantly under stress (or *thinks* it is)?

Rarely do we find ourselves constantly running from a burglar, but physical stress also includes encounters with potentially deadly toxins and pathogens. And these we may face daily through our dietary choices alone. Although the body may not necessarily go into fight-or-flight mode with a pounding heart when it meets a substance or ingredient it doesn't like, it most definitely will experience an immune response. And chronic immune activation and resulting inflammation from such encounters can lead to chronic disease, from heart and brain diseases like Parkinson's, multiple sclerosis, depression, and dementia to autoimmune disorders, ulcerative colitis, and cancer. We'll explore this process in more detail in the next chapter, but understand for now that all manner of disease is rooted in inflammation run amok, and your immune system controls inflammation. How does the microbiome come into play?

It *regulates* or manages the immune response. So it, in turn, takes part in the story of inflammation in your body. Let me break this down a bit more for you.

Although each of us is under constant threat from injurious chemicals and germs, we have a great defense system: immunity. When the immune system is compromised, we quickly fall prey to any number of possible disease-causing agents. Without an adequately functioning immune system, an event as simple as a mosquito bite could conceivably prove fatal. And beyond extrinsic events like insect bites, every part of us is colonized moment to moment by any number of potentially life-threatening organisms that, were it not for an appropriately functioning immune system, could easily render our death. At the same time, it is important to recognize that the immune system functions optimally when it is in balance.

An overactive immune system can lead to such complications as allergies; in a severe case, it can react so wildly that it leads to anaphylactic shock—an extreme reaction that can be deadly. In addition, when the immune system is misdirected, it may fail to recognize normal body proteins as being part of the self and rebel against them. This is the basic mechanism of autoimmune diseases, which are generally treated with aggressive immune-suppressing drugs that often have significant downsides, not the least of which includes changing the array of bacteria in the gut. The immune system is to blame when a transplant patient rejects what is supposed to be a life-saving organ. And it is the immune system that helps the body recognize and eliminate cancerous cells, a process that's occurring right now inside you.

Your gut has its own immune system, the "gut-associated lymphatic tissue" (GALT). It represents 70 to 80 percent of your body's total immune system. This speaks volumes about the importance—and vulnerability—of your gut. If the events that take place in the gut weren't so critical to life, then the majority of your immune system wouldn't have to be there to guard and protect it.

The reason most of your immune system is deployed in your gut is simple: the intestinal wall is the border with the outside world. Aside from skin, it's where your body has the most chances of encountering foreign material and organisms. And it is in constant communication with every other immune system cell in the body. If it meets a problematic substance in the gut, it alerts the rest of the immune system to be on guard.

One of the overarching themes you'll read throughout the book is the importance of retaining the integrity of that delicate intestinal wall, which is only one cell thick. It must remain intact while acting as a conduit for signals between the gut bacteria and the immune system's cells right on the other side. In the words of Dr. Alessio Fasano of Harvard—who lectured on the topic at a 2014 conference, which I attended, that was dedicated solely to the science of the microbiome—these immune cells that receive signals from the gut bacteria are the body's "first responders." In turn, the gut bacteria help keep the immune system vigilant but not in full defense mode. They monitor and "educate" the immune system. This ultimately helps prevent your gut's immune system from inappropriately reacting to foods and triggering autoimmune responses. We'll see in upcoming chapters just how critical the gut-associated lymphatic tissue is in preserving your body's overall health. It's your body's military, on the lookout for any threats coming down the intestinal pipeline that can adversely impact the body all the way up to the brain.

Both human and animal studies show that bad or pathogenic gut bacteria can cause disease, but not just because they are associated with a specific condition. We know that *Helicobacter pylori*, for instance, is responsible for creating ulcers. But it turns out that pathogenic bacteria also interact with the immune system in the gut to cause the release of inflammatory molecules and stress hormones, essentially flipping the switch on our body's stress response system so it thinks we're being preyed upon by a lion. New science is also revealing that bad bacteria can change how we perceive pain; indeed, people with an unhealthy microbiome may be more sensitive to pain.[8]

Good bacteria in the gut do the opposite. They try to minimize the amount and effects of the bad guys while also interacting positively with both the immune and endocrine systems. That is to say, the good bacteria can turn off that chronic immune system response. They can also help keep in check cortisol and adrenaline — the two hormones associated with stress that can wreak havoc on the body when they are continually flowing.

Each large group of gut bacteria has many different strains, and each of these strains may have different effects. The two most common groups of organisms in the gut, representing more than 90 percent of the bacterial population in the colon, are Firmicutes (pronounced fir-MIH-cue-tees) and Bacteroidetes (pronounced BAC-teer-OY-deh-tees). Firmicutes are notorious as "fat-loving" bacteria, for it's been shown that the bacteria in the Firmicutes family are equipped with more enzymes to digest complex carbohydrates, so they are much more efficient at extracting energy (i.e., calories) from food. They also were just recently found to be instrumental in increasing fat absorption.[9] Researchers have discovered that obese people have elevated levels of Firmicutes in their gut flora, compared to lean people, who are dominated more by Bacteroidetes.[10] In fact, the relative proportion of these two groups to each other, the Firmicutes-to-Bacteroidetes (or F/B) ratio, is critical for determining health and risk for illness. What's more, we've just learned that higher levels of Firmicutes actually turn on genes that increase the risk for obesity, diabetes, and even cardiovascular disease.[11] Think of that: Changes in the ratio of these bacteria can change the actual expression of *your* DNA!

The two most studied strains of bacteria today are those of *Bifido-bacterium* and *Lactobacillus*. Don't worry about having to remember these long names. In this book, you'll be hearing about many types of bacteria that have complicated Latin names, but I promise that by the end you'll be able to distinguish among many different strains. Although we can't say for sure yet exactly which strains in which proportions are ideal for optimal health, the general thinking is that variety is key.

I should also point out that the line between "good" and "bad" bacteria isn't as clear as you might assume. Again, overall diversity and the ratios of strains relative to one another are the important factors. In the wrong ratio, certain strains that can have positive effects on health can turn into villains. The notorious bacteria *Escherichia coli*, for instance, produces vitamin K but can cause severe illness. *Helicobacter pylori*, the bacteria I just mentioned that causes peptic ulcers, also helps regulate appetite in a positive way so you don't overeat.

For one more example, consider *Clostridium difficile*, a strain of bacteria that can lead to a life-endangering infection if it's allowed to overgrow. The illness, characterized by intense diarrhea, still kills approximately 14,000 Americans each year; *C. difficile* infections have risen sharply over the last twenty years.[12] Between 1993 and 2005, the number of cases among hospitalized adults tripled; between 2001 and 2005, it more than doubled.[13] Mortality rates have also soared, largely due to the emergence of a mutant, hypervirulent strain.

Normally, all of us as babies had intestines that were colonized with generous amounts of the *C. difficile* bacterium and it caused no problem. It's found in the intestines of up to 63 percent of newborns and even a third of toddlers. But a change in the gut environment, for example through overuse of certain antibiotics, can spur excessive growth of this bacteria, resulting in a life-threatening illness. The good news is that we now have a very effective way to treat such an infection, through the use of other strains of bacteria to restore balance.

You'll learn more about the microbiome and its relationship with the immune system and brain in the upcoming chapters, but this is a good time to jump to the following question: Where do our brotherly bugs originate? In other words, how do they become a part of us?

BABY YOU'RE BORN WITH IT! SORT OF . . .

Much of what we know about the microbiome comes from studying so-called germ-free mice. These are mice that have been altered to not have any gut bacteria, thereby allowing scientists to study the effects of missing microbes or, conversely, exposing them to certain strains and watching what happens. Germ-free lab rats have been shown, for example, to have acute anxiety, an inability to handle stress, chronic gut and general inflammation, and lower levels of an important brain-growth hormone called BDNF (brain-derived neurotrophic factor).[14] But these symptoms can be reversed once the rats are fed a diet rich in *Lactobacillus helveticus* or *Bifidobacterium longum*, two common probiotics.

It is thought that each of us was once germ-free, when we were in our mother's womb, a relatively sterile environment. (I expect this notion to be challenged very soon, for new science is just emerging that suggests the fetus may be exposed to microbes in utero through the placenta, and that the microbiome actually begins there.[15] Stay tuned for more definitive studies on this subject.) The current thinking is that the moment we move through the birth canal and are exposed to organisms in the vagina, our microbiome begins to develop. And while people may not want to picture this in their minds, even the mother's fecal material in the perianal area helps to inoculate the newborn with health-sustaining microorganisms.

In terms of the initial development of a healthy immune system, a significant factor in establishing the "set-point" for inflammation may be an individual's method of birth. It's one of the most influential events in determining the functional outcome of the microbiome. By set-point, I am referring to the body's average or baseline level of inflammation. It helps to think of your set-point as a built-in thermostat that is programmed to a particular temperature. If your set-point is high, such as a thermostat fixed at 78 degrees, overall your general level of inflammation is higher than someone whose set-point is lower. Even though there may be some variations, overall a higher set-point means a higher degree of temperature (inflammation). And as I just mentioned, how you were born affects how your microbiome developed initially, which in turn influenced your innate set-point for inflammation.

Can you change your set-point? Yes—absolutely. Just as you can change your set-point for body weight and body mass index (BMI) through diet and exercise, you can change your set-point for inflammation through basic lifestyle interventions. But before we get to all that, it's important for you to appreciate the power of early life experiences, and how method of birth shapes health risks in a person's life.

Multiple high-profile studies have compared the difference between children born via C-section and those born vaginally.[16] In addition to comparing dominant characteristics of these two groups' microbiomes, they've examined the associated health implications and reached many alarming conclusions. These studies have shown that there's a clear correlation between what colonizes a baby's intestines and what is found in the mother's birth canal. One particularly fascinating study performed by a team of researchers in 2010 revealed that when they used gene sequencing to profile bacterial types from mothers and their newborn babies, they found that infants born vaginally obtained bacterial colonies resembling their own mothers' vaginal microbiome, dominated by beneficial *Lactobacillus*, whereas babies born via C-section acquired colonies similar to those found on the skin's surface, dominated by an abundance of the potentially harmful *Staphylococcus*.[17]

In 2013, the *Canadian Medical Association Journal* included a study that stated the facts bluntly, showing how disruption of the infant's gut microbiota has been linked to many inflammatory and immune problems like allergies, asthma, and even cancer.[18] These researchers highlighted the impact of a baby's birth experience and whether he or she is breast-fed or placed on formula. They rightfully referred to the gut microbiota as a "super organ" with "diverse roles in health and disease." In related commentary about the study, Dr. Rob Knight of the esteemed Knight Lab at the University of Colorado, Boulder, said: "Children born by cesarean delivery or fed with formula may be at increased risk of a variety of conditions later in life; both processes alter the gut microbiota in healthy infants, which could be the mechanism for the increased risk."[19]

What makes *Lactobacillus* so superior is that it creates a slightly acidic environment, which reduces the growth of potentially dangerous bacteria. *Lactobacillus* bacteria are able to utilize milk sugar, or lactose, as a fuel. This enables babies to use lactose from their mother's milk. By and large, infants born by cesarean section may not receive an abundant supply of *Lactobacillus*; instead, they are exposed more to what's lurking around the operating room and on the doctors' and nurses' hands—skin bacteria that tend to be dominated by types that don't impart many benefits. Moreover, as Dr. Martin Blaser describes in his terrific book, *Missing Microbes*, every single woman in America receives antibiotics when giving birth by C-section, and that means that all the infants born surgically start life exposed to a powerful antibiotic—a double whammy.[20]

Dr. Blaser, who directs New York University's Microbiome Program, further points out that a third of infants born in the U.S. today are born by C-section, which reflects a 50 percent increase since 1996. If this trend continues, by 2020 half of the babies born in the U.S. will be delivered surgically. I love how Blaser so eloquently states the facts of the matter: "The fancy names of these bacteria don't matter so much as the notion that the founding populations of microbes found on C-section infants are not those selected by hundreds of thousands of years of human evolution or even longer."[21]

Studies have also proven that vaginally born infants have much higher levels of bifidobacteria, a group of beneficial gut bacteria that help to mature the gut lining more quickly.[22] Surgically born babies, on the other hand, lack this type of good bacteria. One way to think about the birthing process is to understand that it's like giving a newborn a set of instructions for a healthy start to life. It's the last major transmission a baby receives from its mother after being in utero. Babies who arrive via C-section are missing some of these instructions. And they may never either artificially or even through breastfeeding or diet.

The statistics regarding the health consequences of being born through the abdomen as opposed to the vagina are absolutely stunning. Here's a small snapshot of what being born by C-section can entail, based on a large population and rigorously controlled studies:

- A five-fold increased risk of allergies[23]

- Triple the risk of ADHD[24]

- Twice the risk of autism[25]

- An 80 percent increased risk of celiac disease[26]

- A 50 percent increased risk of becoming obese as an adult (and, as we'll see later, being obese is directly correlated with an increased risk of dementia)[27]

- A 70 percent increased risk of type-1 diabetes[28] (and being diabetic more than doubles the risk for dementia)[29]

Let me be clear: C-sections do save lives, and they are medically necessary under certain situations. But most experts, including home-birth midwives and obstetricians who specialize in high-risk births, agree that only a fraction of deliveries need to be done surgically, and yet these operations are often a *choice* now being made by American women.[30] In 2014, a new nationwide study revealed that 26 percent of U.S. mothers delivered via C-section in 2001, and 45 percent of these deliveries were not considered medically indicated.[31] So my concerns revolve squarely around the trend in choosing to have a C-section for reasons that are not necessarily in the interest of the baby or mother. That said, a pregnant woman could have every good intention of giving birth vaginally and then face unexpected circumstances that call for a C-section. She should never feel guilty or fearful that she's jeopardizing her child's future health.

Later in the book I'll provide explicit information, for both expecting mothers and those who've already given birth, on how to compensate for a surgical delivery. There's a lot you can do to support a newborn's developing microbiome and counteract potential negative effects from medical interventions taken during childbirth.

Although it's logical to assume this passing on of microbes from mother to child through the birth canal is unique to mammals, we have evidence that other species do indeed pass on their microbial heritage to their offspring, albeit through different mechanisms.[32] These other species include marine sponges (which evolved 600 million years ago as the first multicellular animals), clams, aphids, cockroaches, whiteflies, stinkbugs, chickens, and turtles. The point is that transmission of microbes from one generation to the next is a fundamental process of life.

THE THREE FORCES WORKING AGAINST YOUR BELLY BUGS

Although you can't change how you were born, how you were initially fed, and what kind of microbiome developed in (and on) you as an infant, the good news is that you still have the power to change, heal, and nourish a healthy microbiome through what you eat, what you're exposed to in the environment, and what kind of lifestyle you lead. By now, you probably have a general sense of what can work against the health of your gut's good bugs. I'll detail all the potential triggers and causes of a sick microbiome later on. But as a primer, let's briefly run through the three strongest forces at work.

- Force #1: Exposure to substances that kill or otherwise adversely change the composition of the bacterial colonies. These include everything from environmental chemicals to certain ingredients in food (e.g., sugar, gluten), water (e.g., chlorine), and drugs like antibiotics.

- Force #2: Lack of nutrients that support healthy, diverse tribes of bacteria and instead favor bad bacteria. I'll share which foods and supplements ensure the health of the microbiome and, in turn, the brain.

- Force: #3: Stress. While it may sound like a cliché to say that stress is bad for your health, I'll explain why it's even worse than we previously thought.

Clearly, some of these are impossible to avoid at all times. There will be situations, for example, when antibiotics are life-saving and necessary. Later on, I'll give you some instructions for handling such situations so you can preserve the health of your gut (or your child's gut as in the case of being prescribed antibiotics for an infection during pregnancy) as much as possible. This will, in turn, help preserve the health and function of your brain.

THE "DIRTY" SECRET ABOUT MODERN PLAGUES

One of the themes of this book is the power of dirt, so to speak. Put another way, there's immense value in being *un*-hygienic. Astonishing new studies show a relationship between our increasingly sterile living environments and incidence of chronic illnesses, from heart disease and autoimmune disorders to cancer and dementia.

At Stanford University's School of Medicine, husband and wife team Erica and Justin Sonnenburg run a lab in the department of microbiology and immunology, where they are focusing on understanding the interactions within the intestinal microbiome and those between gut bacteria and the human host. In particular, they are investigating how a loss of microbial species and diversity in Western civilizations due to diet, use of antibiotics, and overly sanitized conditions may explain why we suffer from rising rates of "Western" diseases, which are not seen nearly as much in traditional, mostly agrarian societies.

In a recent paper, they write convincingly that we may be experiencing an "incompatibility" between our DNA, which has remained relatively stable over the course of human history, and our microbiome, which has experienced dramatic changes in response to our modern lifestyles.[33] They also highlight how our Western diets, which are low in plant fibers that serve as fuel for gut bacteria, result in fewer types of microbes and beneficial byproducts that our gut bacteria produce when they metabolize or ferment our food. We are, in their words, "starving our microbial self," and this may have drastic health consequences. The byproducts, by the way, that our gut bacteria produce help control inflammation as well as our immune system's response — two key factors in all manner of chronic illness. The Sonnenburgs write, "It is possible that the Western microbiota is actually dysbiotic and predisposes individuals to a variety of diseases."[34]

THE WESTERN DIET MAKES FOR A WESTERN MICROBIOME

When you compare the microbiome of children from Africa with that of children from Europe, you find a big difference. The "Western" microbiome significantly lacks diversity, and has more bacteria from the group Firmicutes than the group Bacteroidetes, the two types of bacteria that dominate the gut's ecology. Firmicutes are notoriously good at helping the body extract more calories from food and aiding in the uptake of fats, hence their association with weight gain when they dominate in the gut. Bacteroidetes, on the other hand, don't have this same capacity. So the pattern of higher levels of Firmicutes and lower levels of Bacteroidetes is associated with a greater risk of obesity.[35] It's seen in people from urban areas, while the opposite is more common in people from rural areas.

Another way of seeing the connection between a clean, low-fiber Western lifestyle and incidence of chronic illness is to consider the wealth factor. Do wealthier and cleaner nations have higher rates of, say, Alzheimer's disease? This was demonstrated in some excellent research published in 2013, which was carried out at the University of Cambridge.[36] Dr. Molly Fox and her colleagues assessed 192 countries around the world, looking at two things. First, they examined rates of parasite infestation and diversity of gut bacteria in people from these countries. And second, they reviewed the rate of Alzheimer's disease.

What they found was truly remarkable. In those countries having the least sanitation, the prevalence of Alzheimer's was dramatically reduced. But in countries with higher degrees of sanitation, and therefore lower levels of parasites as well as less diversity of intestinal organisms, Alzheimer's prevalence skyrocketed. In countries where more than 75 percent of people reside in urban areas, such as the United Kingdom and Australia, Alzheimer's rates were 10 percent higher than in countries where less than one tenth of people live in urban areas, such as Nepal and Bangladesh. Their conclusions state, "Based on our analysis, it appears that hygiene is positively associated with Alzheimer's disease risk... variation in hygiene may partly explain global patterns in Alzheimer's disease rates. Microorganism exposure may be inversely related to Alzheimer's disease risk. These results may help predict Alzheimer's disease burden in developing countries where microbial diversity is rapidly diminishing."

In the images on the next page, notice how the countries in the first graphic with the highest levels of parasites, such as Kenya, are depicted in the second graphic as having the lowest rates of Alzheimer's disease.

Now, correlation (like that found in this study) doesn't necessarily indicate causation. Just because attention to hygiene is strongly associated with increased risk of Alzheimer's disease doesn't necessarily mean it causes Alzheimer's disease rates to rise. There are many variables at play when it comes to the development of any given disease, as well as

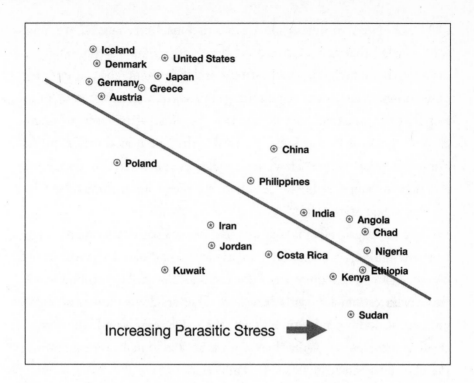

Increasing Parasitic Stress ➡

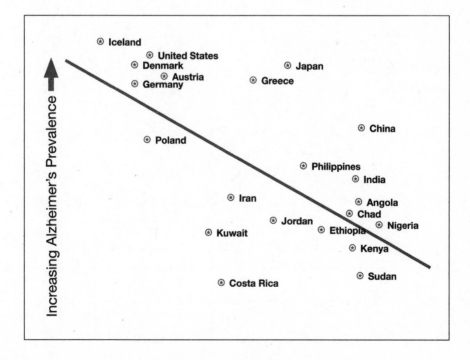

Increasing Alzheimer's Prevalence

incidence of certain illnesses in various nations. But, that said, we must acknowledge that the evidence continues to mount to the extent it makes it hard to ignore such strong and consistent correlations. It's observational, but deductive reasoning compels us to at least consider the fact that our microbiome is factoring—big time—into risk for many chronic diseases. It also forces us to ask the question that Dr. Justin Sonnenburg has posed: "How much influence do bacteria have over us? Are humans simply elaborate vessels for the propagation of microbes?"[37]

A good question indeed.

The inescapable fact is that we have evolved with these microorganisms over millions of years. They are as much a part of our survival as our own cells are. We require them for life and health. Unfortunately, we treat the intestinal flora with disrespect. They are doing vital work under hazardous conditions. It's time to give them due regards and take care of them as they deserve. Only then will we be able to make serious, meaningful headway against our modern afflictions.

CHAPTER 2

Belly and Brain on Fire

The New Science of Inflammation

KNOWING WHAT I KNOW TODAY about the role of diet in the risk of disease and progression of an illness, I am deeply saddened when I think of my father, who was once a brilliant neurosurgeon, trained at the prestigious Lahey Clinic in Massachusetts, and who now resides in an assisted-living facility located across the parking lot from my office. His brain has been ravaged by Alzheimer's disease. More often than not, he doesn't recognize me and still thinks he's practicing medicine, though he retired more than twenty-five years ago.

I sometimes wonder, what could he have done differently to prevent this fate? What could *any* of my patients do to prevent this fate? The same questions go through my head as those in the families I counsel who are struggling with a tragic diagnosis in a loved one: *Why did this happen? What did he or she do wrong? When did it start? Could we have averted this somehow?* And then I remind myself of the key process in the body that has everything to do with brain disease: inflammation.

What does inflammation have to do with the microbiome? That's what we're going to explore in this chapter. I'm going to couch this discussion within the context of Alzheimer's disease, arguably the most dreaded neurological ailment of all, which affects some 5.4 million Americans. This will help you understand the indelible connection between the state of your gut's microbial community and the fate of your brain.

BOONDOGGLE OF THE 21ST CENTURY

In 2014, I wrote an online article titled "Why We Can and Must Focus on Preventing Alzheimer's," following an announcement in the *New York Times* about a new partnership forged among the NIH, ten pharmaceutical companies, and seven nonprofit organizations.[1,2] Their mission is dedicated to developing drugs to treat Alzheimer's disease, among other illnesses. No question, this five-year, $230 million effort seems noble at first, but I declared, "the ultimate motivation for this seemingly ecumenical event is suspect."

Alzheimer's disease is expensive. The $200 billion annual price tag I mentioned in the introduction doesn't include the emotional expense borne by family members whose lives are somberly compromised by this disease, sometimes for a long time. As the *Times* article divulged, drug companies "have invested staggering amounts of money in developing drugs to treat Alzheimer's disease, for example, but again and again the medications have failed in testing." That same year, the *New England Journal of Medicine* reported that two of the promising drug candidates for treating Alzheimer's disease had failed to provide any meaningful benefit.[3,4]

Adding to this disturbing report came another published in the *Journal of the American Medical Association* showing that the drug memantine, currently approved by the Food and Drug Administration (FDA) for treating moderate to severe Alzheimer's disease, was not only ineffective but also associated with *more* decline in patients' functionality when compared to a placebo.[5]

The reason we should temper our support for this collaboration is that it represents a "perversion of priority." As I wrote in the article, "Those who would be most enthusiastic about these seemingly forthright liaisons and monetary expenditures may be focused on the development of a blockbuster magic bullet for the treatment of Alzheimer's disease for reasons that are less invested in alleviating suffering and more invested in financial outcome." Harsh, I know. But I meant it to be a clarion call to switch gears and explore another option.

Rather than paying so much attention (and money) to developing treatments for Alzheimer's disease (or any neurodegenerative ailment, for that matter), we must focus on educating people about preventive efforts. These preventive strategies are already well documented in high-profile scientific literature and can have a radical impact in reducing the incidences of the neurodegenerative illness. Medical researchers already have knowledge that, if implemented, could slash the number of new Alzheimer's patients here in the U.S. by more than half. And when you consider that the number of people stricken with Alzheimer's is predicted to double by the year 2030, spreading the word about this information should be top priority.[6]

Economic and marketplace realities unfortunately are formidable barriers to overcome. Few, if any, opportunities exist to monetize such nonproprietary interventions like diet and exercise, which, among other lifestyle strategies, are well known to play important roles in both brain degeneration and, on the other hand, preservation.

Here's one fine example of a major lifestyle factor: Our best medical journals are now brimming with high-profile, rigorous studies that show a stunning correlation between high blood sugar and risk for dementia. As reported in the *New England Journal of Medicine* in 2013, even slight elevations of blood sugar that are far below the diabetes range have been shown to significantly increase the risk for the development of untreatable dementia.[7] Researchers from the University of Washington evaluated a group of more than 2,000 individuals whose average age was 76 years. At the beginning of the study, they measured their fasting blood sugar levels, and then followed these individuals for about seven years. Some of the people developed dementia over that time period. What the researchers discovered was that there was a direct correlation between blood sugar levels at the start of the study and risk for developing dementia. It's important to understand that these individuals were not diabetic; they had blood sugar levels well below the threshold for a diagnosis of diabetes.

Blood sugar directly reflects dietary choices; eat too many refined sugars and carbs and you'll have a hard time controlling your blood sugar. I'll describe the link between blood sugar balance and risk for dementia shortly, but suffice it to say this kind of knowledge provides a significant leverage point that can move the needle on cognitive health.

Further, in 2013 the *Journal of Neurology, Neurosurgery and Psychiatry* published a study showing that elderly people who added more fat, in the form of olive oil or mixed nuts, to their diets maintained their cognitive function much better over a six-year period than people who ate a low-fat diet.[8] The potential implications of studies like these are poised to revolutionize medicine as we know it. But sadly, disease prevention through non-invasive, simple daily lifestyle choices lacks the seeming heroism of bold, pharmaceutical-based interventions. It's time that we take a new road and champion preventive medicine, especially for brain health. We can afford to do no less. Rather than expending huge resources to find the cow after the barn door has been left open, maybe we should see about keeping the barn door closed in the first place. And that metaphorical barn door has a lot to do with the state of your microbiome. To understand this connection, let's first explore the role of inflammation, then circle back to the underlying power of your gut bacteria.

INFLAMMATION: THE COMMON DENOMINATOR

We are all familiar with inflammation. The word itself comes from the Latin verb *inflammare*, which means "to kindle" or "to set on fire." Inflamed flesh is burning up—and not in a good way. An inflammatory cascade might include the redness, heat, and swelling that accompanies an insect bite or the pain you experience with a sore throat or sprained ankle. We generally accept the notion that a bite or scrape to the skin is going to be painful because of inflammation. But inflammation is involved in far more disease processes than you can possibly imagine. Indeed, it is the crux of the body's healing response, bringing more immune activity to a place of injury or infection. But when inflammation persists or serves no purpose, deep inside the body and through systemic pathways, it causes illness. In fact, it's implicated in such diverse conditions as obesity, diabetes, cancer, depression, autism, asthma, arthritis, coronary artery disease, multiple sclerosis, and even Parkinson's and Alzheimer's disease.

Let's look at Alzheimer's in particular. Inflammation is exactly what is happening in the brain of a patient with Alzheimer's disease. This inflammation may be difficult to spot, I realize, because when the brain is inflamed we don't see what we think of as the normal signs of inflammation, such as pain and swelling. The brain, although able to perceive pain anywhere in the body, doesn't itself have pain receptors and therefore cannot register the fact that it's up in smoke. Nonetheless, scientific research has, for the past several decades, clearly demonstrated over and over again that inflammation is a fundamental process that underlies the development of Alzheimer's disease.[9]

A multitude of biochemicals are related to inflammation both in the brain and throughout the body. In Alzheimer's patients, biochemicals that indicate that inflammation is occurring—inflammatory markers— are elevated and can even be used to *predict* cognitive decline and the development of dementia. Among the most famous of these biochemicals are the cytokines, small proteins released by cells that affect the behavior of other cells and are often important participants in the inflammatory process. C-reactive protein, interleukin six (IL-6), and tumor necrosis factor alpha (TNF-α) are all cytokines. We now have the ability to image the brain in ways that allow us to see these inflammatory chemicals in action, so we can identify direct correlations between the degree of inflammation and the degree of cognitive impairment.

TNF-α in particular seems to play an important role in inflammation throughout the body, and in addition to being elevated in the blood of Alzheimer's patients, it's been found to be elevated in a variety of other inflammatory conditions including psoriasis, rheumatoid arthritis, cardiovascular disease, Crohn's disease, and asthma.[10, 11] So important is the role of TNF-α in these conditions that pharmaceutical companies are investing huge sums of money to try to develop ways of reducing it. The global market for TNF inhibitors today exceeds $20 billion annually.[12]

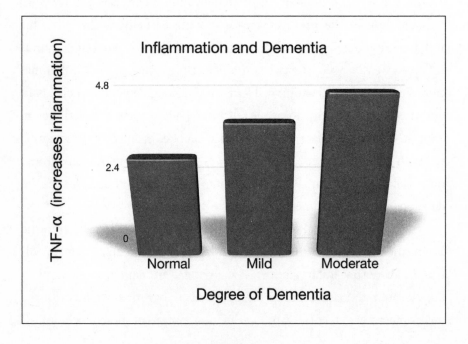

In some people, specific genes can naturally increase inflammation, and they can further raise one's risk for developing diseases rooted in inflammation.[13] But genetic factors are far from the whole story. You can do a lot to influence the expression of your genes, from turning off or suppressing "bad" genes to flipping the switch on "good" genes that will help assure your health.

In *Grain Brain* I explored in-depth one of the most influential and fundamental ways one can support the expression of those good genes while suppressing the bad and, in turn, keep inflammation in check when it's not needed for survival: by maintaining healthful blood sugar levels. Elevated blood sugar stirs up inflammation in the bloodstream, as excess sugar can be toxic if it's not swept up and used by cells. It also triggers a reaction called glycation — the biological process by which sugar binds to proteins and certain fats, resulting in deformed molecules that don't function well. These sugar proteins are technically called advanced glycation end products (AGEs). The body does not recognize AGEs as normal, so they set off inflammatory reactions. In the brain, sugar molecules and brain proteins combine to produce lethal new structures that contribute to the degeneration of the brain and its functioning.

The relationship between poor blood sugar control and Alzheimer's disease in particular is so strong that researchers are now calling Alzheimer's disease type-3 diabetes.[14] Although the studies documenting this phenomenon go back about ten years now, newer science is further crystallizing the big picture. We are finding out that alterations in the gut microbiota pave the way for the development of diabetes and proliferation of AGEs and therefore increase the risk for Alzheimer's disease. I'll detail how this is possible in chapter 4, but here's a quick primer.

In 2012, the journal *Nature* published a study showing that people with type 2 diabetes suffered from bacterial imbalances (dysbiosis) in their gut.[15] These imbalances caused them to lack important byproducts from the gut bacteria that are needed to maintain the health of cells in the digestive system. Bear in mind that people who have type 2 diabetes are under a lot of metabolic stress because their bodies cannot transport glucose successfully from the bloodstream into their cells. And in areas of the body that don't have a glucose transport system, such as the nerves and brain, scientists can identify other forms of metabolic stress such as those AGEs, which can result in conditions including peripheral neuropathy (weakness, numbness, and pain caused by damaged nerves), and damage to blood vessels and brain function.

This discovery has been groundbreaking in my world. To know that at the center of the cascade of events leading to diabetes and brain disease is a disrupted gut community is, at least to me, staggering. I love how a group of Chinese researchers recently explained the facts of the matter in a report published in the esteemed *Food Science and Human Wellness* journal:[16]

[G]reat progress has been made in the field of the resident microbiota in type-2 diabetes in recent years. Microbiota contribute not only to low-level inflammation in the onset of type-2 diabetes, but also to the further development of type-2 diabetes through inflammatory components. It has also been extended to various type-2 diabetes related complications, including diabetic retinopathy, kidney toxicity, atherosclerosis, hypertension, diabetic foot ulcers, cystic fibrosis and Alzheimer's disease. These studies together support the crucial role of microbiota in maintaining the intestinal barrier integrity, sustaining a normal metabolic homeostasis, protecting the host from infection by pathogens, enhancing host defense systems and even influencing the nervous system in type-2 diabetes.

The researchers went on to discuss the influential role of dietary choices in changing the microbiota for the better and reducing risk for these conditions. They also pointed out that various herbs and supplements with known anti-diabetic properties work to control blood sugar *through the microbiome.* In other words, they may not necessarily be directly affecting insulin and glucose; rather, they are positively affecting the microbiome. For example, the traditional Chinese herbal components berberine and ginseng, as well as the compounds found in tea, coffee, wine, and chocolate have anti-diabetic qualities through their effects on gut bacteria. These compounds either change the composition of gut bacteria for the better or are metabolized by the gut bacteria before being absorbed into the body. After thousands of years, ancient Chinese herbal practices are finally getting the explanation they deserve. It's the gut bugs that are making use of these herbal compounds first so we can benefit from them.

Dr. James M. Hill is a senior scientific investigator and professor of neuroscience at Louisiana State University School of Medicine. His laboratory is among many high-tech labs connecting the dots between the gut's microbiome and the risk for brain disease. He recently published a report outlining the multiple ways in which the brain and its functioning are influenced by what goes on in the gut.[17] In his studies using mouse models, he's explored how good gut bacteria are capable of producing important brain chemicals like BDNF, gamma-amino butyric acid (GABA), and glutamate. And levels of these important chemicals directly reflect what goes on in terms of gut bacteria; when researchers disrupt gut bacteria in mice, they not only observe behavioral changes in the mice, but also calculate changes in the volume of these chemicals.

Previously, I described brain-derived neurotrophic factor as a critical brain-growth protein. BDNF is involved in neurogenesis, the process by which new neurons are created. BDNF also protects existing neurons, ensuring their survival and encouraging connections, or synapses, between them. This synapse formation is essential for thinking, learning, and higher levels of brain function. Decreased levels of BDNF are found in a panoply of neurological conditions, including Alzheimer's, epilepsy, anorexia nervosa, depression, schizophrenia, and obsessive-compulsive disorder. And while we know that BDNF can be increased through aerobic exercise as well as by consuming the omega-3 fat DHA, we are now learning that this critically important brain chemical is vitally dependent on the balance of bacteria that live within the gut.

In the American Medical Association's journal *JAMA Neurology*, a fascinating report by a team at Boston University School of Medicine, published in November 2013, revealed how blood levels of BDNF relate to risk for developing dementia.[18] The study culled information from the now-famous Framingham Heart Study, one of the largest epidemiological studies ever performed, to look at blood levels of BDNF in a group of 2,131 adults. These individuals were free of dementia at the start and were followed for up to 10 years.

What these Boston University researchers found was that those individuals at the beginning of the study who had the highest levels of BDNF had less than half the risk of dementia compared to those with the lowest BDNF levels. They stated that BDNF "may also be reduced in healthy people who are destined to develop dementia or Alzheimer's disease." The researchers concluded the obvious: "Our findings suggest a role for BDNF in the biology and possibly in the prevention of dementia and Alzheimer's disease."[19]

GABA, another important chemical manufactured by the gut bacteria, is an amino acid that serves as a neurotransmitter in the central nervous system. It's the main chemical messenger in your brain that calms down nerve activity by inhibiting transmissions and normalizing brain waves. In other words, GABA returns the nervous system to a more stable state so you can weather stress better. In 2012, researchers at Baylor College of Medicine and Texas Children's Hospital identified a strain of bifidobacteria that secretes large amounts of GABA, suggesting that it may play a role in preventing or treating not just brain disorders but inflammatory bowel disorders such as Crohn's disease.[20] Because GABA mutes neuronal activity, it keeps in check anxiety — anxiety, of course, being a common trigger to gastrointestinal (GI) disorders rooted in inflammation.

Glutamate, yet another vital neurotransmitter that is produced by the gut bacteria, is involved in most aspects of normal brain function, including cognition, learning, and memory. It's abundant in a healthy brain. A slew of neurological challenges, from anxiety and behavioral deficits to depression and Alzheimer's disease, have been attributed to a lack of GABA and glutamate.

One of the most important takeaways from the new research on the connection between microbes and brain health is that "disruption" isn't just about having a misbalanced microbiome, in which the thugs outnumber and trample on the good guys, triggering inflammation and robbing the body of vital materials produced by those good guys. In millions of people today, the gut is largely disrupted by increased intestinal permeability, which fuels a continuous state of low-grade inflammation. Let me break this down for you.

THE PERILS OF A LEAKY GUT

Your gastrointestinal tract, from the esophagus to the anus, is lined with one single layer of epithelial cells. This cellular layer represents a critical interface between you and your environment ("inside" vs. "outside"). In fact, all of the body's mucosal surfaces, including those of the eyes, nose, throat, and gastrointestinal tract, are a large point of entry for various pathogens, so they must be well protected by the body. (These surfaces are lined by a mucous membrane, a type of tissue that secrets mucus, hence the term *mucosal*.) The intestinal lining, the largest mucosal surface, has three main functions. First, it serves as the vehicle or mechanism by which you obtain nutrients from the foods you eat. Second, it blocks the entrance into the bloodstream of potentially harmful particles, chemicals, bacteria, and other organisms that can pose a threat to your health. Third, it contains chemicals called immunoglobulins that bind to bacteria and foreign proteins to prevent them from attaching to your gut's lining. These chemicals are antibodies that are secreted from immune system cells on the other side of the gut lining and that are transported into the gut via the intestinal wall. This ultimately allows pathogenic organisms and proteins to move on and be excreted.

There are two pathways that the body uses to absorb nutrients from the gut. Using the transcellular pathway, nutrients move through the epithelial cells; and using the paracellular pathway, nutrients pass *between* the epithelial cells. The connection between cells, called a tight junction, is an intricate and highly regulated affair. When we are talking about permeability issues in the gut, or the so-called "leaky gut," we are referring to problems in the competency of these tight junctions, which measure between 10 to 15 Å (Å is the abbreviation for *angstrom*, a unit so small that the only way to picture it is to think of a microscopic space millions of times smaller than the head of a pin; it's much smaller than a typical virus or bacterium). If the junctions aren't working properly, they fail to appropriately police what should be allowed to pass (nutrients) or kept out (potential threats). As the gatekeepers, these junctions determine, to a large extent, the set-point of inflammation — your body's baseline level of inflammation at any given time. It's well documented now that when your intestinal barrier is compromised, you are susceptible — through increased inflammation — to a spectrum of health challenges, including rheumatoid arthritis, food allergies, asthma, eczema, celiac disease, inflammatory bowel disease, HIV, cystic fibrosis, diabetes, autism, Alzheimer's, and Parkinson's.[21]

It's hard to imagine that we would ever want our guts to be leaky, but there are times when this is actually helpful. Certain gut infections, like cholera, caused by the bacteria *Vibrio cholerae*, are characterized by increased leakiness of the bowel *in the other direction*, basically allowing more fluid to enter the gut from the bloodstream, presumably to help dilute the organism and its toxin. This ultimately allows the body to purge the nasty germ through the diarrhea that is so aggressive in this illness.

Interestingly enough, it is exactly this model—the increased permeability of the gut lining that occurs with cholera—that allowed Dr. Alessio Fasano of Harvard to identify the now-established relationship among gluten consumption, increased gut permeability, and widespread inflammation throughout the body.[22] I've had the opportunity to hear Dr. Fasano lecture on this topic a few times. Several years ago he shared the influence of serendipity in his career. He had been researching a way to develop a vaccine for cholera when he accidentally came across this surprising connection, adding a new chapter to the science textbooks about leaky guts, gluten, and inflammation. Proof that research can have unintended revelations.

The perils of a leaky gut begin to seem even more monumental, for new science is telling us that the inflammation brought on by a loss of gut integrity can lead to leaky brains. We've long assumed that somehow the brain is fully insulated and protected from what goes on in the rest of the body, as if it were an untouchable sanctuary. You've probably heard about the highly protective, fortified portal keeping bad things out of the brain: the blood-brain barrier. In years past we used to think of this barrier as an impenetrable wall keeping everything out that could pose as a threat. It has just recently become clear, however, that many substances can threaten the integrity of the blood-brain barrier, letting inside various molecules that may spell trouble, including proteins, viruses, and even bacteria that would normally have been excluded.[23] Think about it: Changes in your gut's environment can undermine the brain's ability to protect itself against potentially toxic invaders.

What's even more alarming is Dr. Fasano's recent discovery that not only is there increased gut permeability when the gut is exposed to gliadin, a protein found in gluten, but in fact the blood-brain barrier also becomes more permeable in response to gliadin exposure.[24] It's as if one door mistakenly opened leads to the opening of another door. Intruders galore.

A question you might be asking at this point is this: How can you test for a leaky gut? Every day I perform simple blood tests on patients to help me get a sense of their gut lining's integrity. I use what's called the Cyrex Array 2, which offers the most sophisticated screening tests on the market today. The array, by Cyrex Labs (www.CyrexLabs.com), measures antibodies produced by the immune system when it is confronted by a molecule called LPS, short for *lipopolysaccharide*. No conversation about the microbiome, inflammation, and brain health can exclude the impact of this molecule.

LPS: THE INCENDIARY DEVICE

If there were ever a clear biological villain that flips on inflammatory pathways in the body, it would be lipopolysaccharide. It is a combination of lipid (fat) and sugars and is a major component of the outer membrane of certain bacteria. In addition to providing a lot of the structural integrity of the bacteria, LPS also protects these bacteria from being digested by bile salts from the gallbladder. LPS-protected bacteria, which are called Gram-negative bacteria—that is, a class of bacteria that do not retain the purple stain used in the Gram staining method used to differentiate bacteria—are normally abundant in the gut, representing as much as 50 to 70 percent of the intestinal flora. We've long known that LPS (which is classed as an "endotoxin," meaning a toxin that comes from within the bacteria) induces a violent inflammatory response in animals if it finds its way into the bloodstream.

LPS is used experimentally in research to instantly create inflammation in laboratory studies. Animal models that are used for such diverse conditions as Alzheimer's disease, multiple sclerosis, inflammatory bowel disorders, diabetes, Parkinson's disease, amyotrophic lateral sclerosis (ALS), rheumatoid arthritis, lupus, depression, and even autism employ LPS because of its ability to quickly push that inflammatory button in the body. This ultimately allows researchers to study these ailments and examine their relationship to inflammation. Human studies show that elevated markers of LPS are seen in many of these conditions.

Normally, LPS is blocked from the bloodstream by the tight junctions that exist between the cells lining the intestine. But, as you can imagine, when those junctions are compromised and the lining becomes leaky or permeable, LPS goes into circulation and can fuel inflammation and inflict damage. So LPS levels in the blood are indicative not only of inflammation in general but also of leakiness of the gut.

In one of the most alarming studies ever done on LPS, grad student Marielle Suzanne Kahn and her colleagues at Texas Christian University showed that injections of LPS into laboratory animals' bodies (not brains) led to overwhelming learning deficits.[25] In addition, these animals developed elevated levels of beta-amyloid in their hippocampus, the brain's memory center. Beta-amyloid is a protein that is strongly implicated in Alzheimer's disease pathology. Researchers are now investigating ways that beta-amyloid can be reduced in the brain or even prevented from forming.

Bottom line: Elevated LPS in the blood could be a big contributor to the increased beta-amyloid in the brain that's so characteristic of Alzheimer's disease. Other studies have demonstrated that mice who receive injections of LPS in their abdomens experience severe memory problems.[26, 27] LPS has also been shown to decrease production of BDNF.[28] Moreover, we now have evidence that there's *three times as much* LPS in the plasma of Alzheimer's patients as in healthy controls.[29] This is powerful information that once again speaks to the gut-brain connection and the impact of inflammation and gut permeability. It's a given that we all have LPS in our guts because it's an important structural component in a lot of the bacteria there, but it shouldn't be a given that it ends up in the bloodstream, where it can be quite destructive.

ALS, also known as Lou Gehrig's disease, is a devastating, almost universally fatal condition for which there is no cure and just one (only modestly effective) FDA-approved drug. It affects more than 30,000

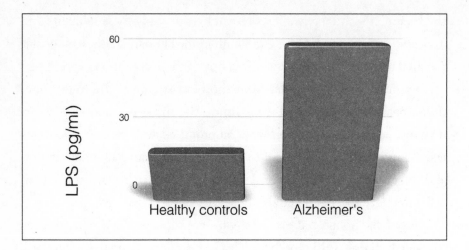

Americans. Research is now looking at the role of LPS and gut permeability in this disease. Not only are there higher levels of LPS in the plasma of ALS patients, but the level of LPS directly correlates to the severity of the illness. This new data has led some experts to wonder if a chief instigator of ALS isn't in the brain or spinal cord, but in the gut. In other words, researchers may have been looking in the wrong place all these years. The evidence against LPS and the inflammation it causes is so incriminating that scientists at the University of San Francisco have stated that this knowledge may "represent novel targets for therapeutic intervention in patients with ALS."[30]

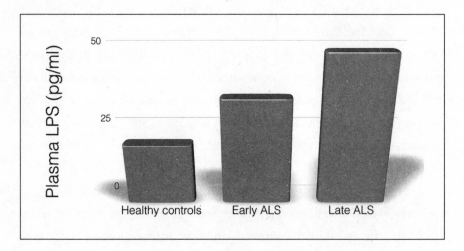

One more example showing the power of LPS: Dr. Christopher Forsyth and his colleagues at Rush University Medical Center in Chicago have explored LPS and intestinal permeability with regard to Parkinson's disease, and they have indeed found direct correlations.[31] Patients with Parkinson's disease show much higher levels of LPS than healthy controls. And in the next chapter, we'll see how the latest science on depression shows that elevated LPS is among the most villainous suspects in triggering the mood disorder.

BRAIN HEALTH BEGINS IN THE GUT

So you should be able to draw the same conclusion I'm going to make. We really have to pay attention to how our gutsy tribes are fed and nurtured. We also have to ensure the integrity of the gut lining. In my previous book, I outlined the primary instigators of inflammation in the body that can interfere with neurological function and brain health—ubiquitous ingredients like gluten and sugar, and a lack of antidotes such as healthy fats, exercise, and restful sleep. But now we have more science to show that the story doesn't just start with an inflammatory response to bread and blintzes. It starts with an upset microbiome and the disastrous effects of molecules like LPS that go rogue once in circulation.

As you'll be learning more about in upcoming chapters, factors such as antibiotics and other medications, chlorinated water, certain foods, and even stress all play a part in determining the diversity and balance of the gut bacteria and, therefore, the set-point of inflammation. Not only do gut microbes influence the environment in your body, but they contribute to that environment by producing certain chemicals that affect the health of the brain and entire nervous system. They determine the strength and fortitude of your gut wall. And they can even produce various vitamins that are essential to brain health, including B12. It's well substantiated that low levels of B12 are a huge risk factor for dementia, not to mention other neurological challenges such as depression.[32] I can't tell you how many times I've seen remarkable improvements in a patient's clinical depression just through B12 supplementation. Research shows that B12 deficiency here in America affects 10 to 15 percent of people over the age of sixty[33] and may well have to do with changes in the gut bacteria as a consequence of poor diet and the medications they take in an attempt to remain healthy. The connection is straightforward: B12 synthesis in the body occurs primarily in the small intestine, where gut bacteria manufacture it using cobalt and other nutrients. Although vitamin B12 can be obtained from the diet, mostly from animal foods including fish, meat, poultry, and eggs, some of the B12 that gets absorbed in the gut to meet your daily requirements comes from those bacterial factories.

I can't reiterate this enough: The health and variety of your belly's bugs directly depend on the foods that you eat. Foods that are high in fiber, which provide fuel to the gut bacteria, and reduced in refined sugars support a robust mélange of bacterial species, which helps maintain the integrity of the gut wall, keep blood sugar in check, reduce inflammation, and manufacture all those important substances and molecules critical for brain health and function. Moreover, there's a big difference between fats that fuel inflammation and fats that help control inflammation. Omega-6 fats dominate in the Western diet today; these are the pro-inflammatory fats found in many vegetable oils that have been linked to an increased risk for brain disorders as well as heart trouble. Omega-3 fats, on the other hand—such as the fats found in olive oil, fish, flaxseed, and wild grass-fed animals—boost brain function, help stamp out inflammation, and can actually counterbalance the detrimental effects of the omega-6 fats. Anthropological research reveals that our hunter-gatherer ancestors consumed omega-6 and omega-3 fats in a ratio of roughly 1:1.[34] Today we consume an astronomical ten to twenty-five times more omega-6 fats than those ancestors did.

Let's briefly turn to the notion of coffee as protective of the brain, as this will further convince you of the power of your dietary choices in light of your gut bacteria. A recent publication in the *Journal of Alzheimer's Disease* revealed an impressive risk reduction for the development of the disease in people who drink coffee. The study, carried out in Finland in collaboration with the Karolinska Institute, followed 1,409 individuals aged 65 to 79 years for an average of 21 years.[35] People who drank between zero and two cups daily were characterized as being "low" coffee drinkers. Those who drank between three and five cups were deemed "moderate," and those who downed more than five cups a day were placed in the "high" category. Moderate drinkers at midlife showed an incredible 65 percent decreased risk for developing Alzheimer's in comparison to low drinkers. (Although the people who drank more than five cups a day also were at reduced risk of dementia, not enough people comprised this group to draw statistically significant conclusions.) Lead researcher Dr. Miia Kivipelto, professor of Clinical Geriatric Epidemiology at Karolinska, commented on her study by stating, "Given the large amount of coffee consumption globally, the results might have important implications for the prevention of or delay the onset of dementia/Alzheimer's disease. The findings need to be confirmed by other studies, but it opens the possibility that dietary interventions could modify the risk of dementia/Alzheimer's disease."[36]

I'd take this a step further. Researchers are just beginning to unravel the brain-protective attributes of coffee, and the latest research plainly demonstrates that it happens at the level of the microbiome. The laboratory research is now extensive, in fact, and unambiguously shows that—through the workings of the belly's bugs—coffee reduces the risks of type-2 diabetes, strokes, Alzheimer's disease, Parkinson's disease, and even cancer and cardiovascular disease.[37, 38] It does this through an array of mechanisms that include the gut bacteria.[39] For starters, intestinal bacteria can easily digest the coffee-bean fiber that remains in the brewed liquid, extracting its energy for their own growth and health. It also has been shown to reduce the ratio of Firmicutes bacteria to Bacteroidetes bacteria, and later on we'll see how this shift in ratio is associated with reduced risk for diabetes and obesity and, therefore, reduced inflammation as well. What's more, we also understand that coffee is a rich source of polyphenols, molecules with known healthful properties. They are the most abundant antioxidants in the human diet. It has been estimated that we consume as much as 1 gram of polyphenols each day, which is about ten times higher than daily consumption of vitamin C and 100 times higher than our daily intake of vitamins E and A. Polyphenols are not only found in coffee; they permeate red wine as well as other foods and have become a major focus of research.

But here's the crux of the matter: The ability of your body to extract and use the polyphenols you consume is dictated largely by the gut bacteria. Those bugs once again take center stage in coordinating your biology for the benefit of your health. In order to fully gain the health benefits of polyphenols from the foods you eat, you need a healthy microbiome.

THE TOP 3 WAYS YOUR GUTSY FRIENDS REDUCE YOUR RISK OF BRAIN DISEASE

1. They help control inflammation. The balance and diversity of gut bacteria regulates how much inflammation occurs in the body. Healthy levels of a variety of good bacteria limit the production of inflammatory chemicals in the body and in the brain. Inflammation, as you already know, is the basis for degenerative conditions in the human body, including diabetes, cancer, coronary heart disease, and Alzheimer's disease.

2. They bolster the intestinal wall's integrity and prevent gut permeability. A leaky gut brought on by an imbalance of gut bacteria allows various proteins normally found in the gut to make their way through the gut wall and challenge the immune system. This scenario turns on an immune response that again leads to inflammation. We now recognize that a variety of factors increase gut permeability, including certain medications, pathogenic bacteria, stress, environmental toxins, elevated blood sugar, and ingredients like gluten.

3. They produce important chemicals for brain health, including BDNF, various vitamins such as B12, and even neurotransmitters like gluta-mate and GABA. They also ferment certain food-borne compounds like polyphenols into smaller anti-inflammatories so they can be absorbed into the bloodstream and ultimately protect the brain.

INFLAMMATION, THE GUT, AND THE MIGHTY MITOCHONDRIA

To bring the conversation about inflammation full circle, we must take a closer look at how our mitochondria serve us. These are the tiny organ-elles, found in all cells except red blood cells, that generate chemical energy in the form of ATP (adenosine triphosphate). They have their own DNA, and the current thinking is that they originated from bacteria—they were once free-living bacteria that ultimately took up residence within our cells and provided our cells the benefit of producing energy. Like bacterial DNA, the DNA of the mitochondria is arranged in a circle, quite unlike the genetic material found within the nucleus of the cell.

We now recognize that these intracellular organelles do far more than simply make energy. Mitochondria exert significant control over nuclear DNA. Given their bacterial origin and their unique DNA, mito-chondria should be considered part of the human microbiome. Healthy mitochondria make for a healthy human. And we now know, for instance, that they play a key role in degenerative diseases such as Alzheimer's, Parkinson's, and even cancer.

First observed by the German doctor Carl Benda in 1897, these intracellular particles appeared as tiny threadlike grains. Hence the name *mitochondria*, derived from the Greek *mitos*, meaning "thread," and *chondrin*, meaning "grain." (As an aside, while the nucleus of the cell contains exactly two copies of its DNA, the mitochondria may have anywhere from 5 to 10 copies of its DNA.)

But it wasn't until 1949 that the role of mitochondria as cellular powerhouse was fully explained by two American scientists, Eugene Kennedy and Albert Lehninger. Basically, these organelles are able to use carbohydrate fuel and convert it to energy that powers most cell functions. The energy produced by this reaction is called oxidative metabolism because oxygen is used up in the process, as it is in a fire. But mitochondrial respiration differs from a fire in that rather than releasing energy in an uncontrolled reaction, mitochondrial energy is stored in a unique molecular form called ATP. Energy-rich ATP can then be delivered throughout the cell, releasing energy on demand in the presence of specific enzymes. Individual cells of the brain, skeletal muscle, heart, kidney, and liver may contain thousands of mitochondria each, to the extent that in some cells, up to 40 percent of the material is made up of mitochondria. According to Professor Enzo Nisoli of the University of Milan, you and I each possess more than ten million billion mitochondria, making up a full 10 percent of our body weight.[40]

A fundamental fact to understand here is that the use of oxygen in the process of producing energy provides a high level of efficiency. While cells do have the ability to utilize other chemical pathways to produce ATP in the absence of oxygen, this process, anaerobic metabolism, is only 1/18 as efficient as oxidative metabolism. But with the use of oxygen comes a price.

An important byproduct of the work done by mitochondria is the production of chemicals, related to oxygen, called reactive oxygen species (ROS). ROS are more commonly known as free radicals. (In a strict scientific sense, the term "free radicals" refers not only to reactive oxygen species, but also a similarly reactive family of radicals, reactive nitrogen species. For purposes of simplification, and as has become the norm in nonscientific publications, we use the term *free radicals* to refer to reactive oxygen species.)

Most everyone is familiar with the term *free radicals* today, for they've been widely described in lay literature, from beauty magazines to advertisements for anti-aging skincare products. Although they are often demonized for the negative effects they can have in the body, free radicals have a positive role in human physiology in a number of ways. They take part in regulating apoptosis, the process by which cells undergo self-destruction (suicide). While it may seem puzzling at first as to why cellular suicide should be looked upon as a favorable event, apoptosis is a critical and necessary cellular function. The term *apoptosis* was first ascribed to Hippocrates and initially taken to mean "the falling off of the leaves." But it was not until a publication in the *British Journal of Cancer* in 1972 by Alastair R. Currie that the term gained traction in the scientific community. Thereafter, researchers used the word to describe the process by which cells are intentionally eliminated.

Without apoptosis, for example, we wouldn't have individual fingers, for it's this very process by which our digits can take shape from the limb buds during our embryological development, thus allowing our hands to form from what initially appear as mittens. Apoptosis is critically important, as it allows our body to rid itself of the multitude of cancer cells that appear spontaneously within us. Each day ten billion cells are terminated to make way for newer, healthier cells. And free radicals created by mitochondria during the process of energy production play a key role in this process.

As with so many things in life, apoptosis does have its dark side. While there are many situations in which activating the demolishing genes of a cell is a good thing, when mitochondrial function becomes impaired, cellular suicide can be induced in otherwise normal, healthy cells. In fact, this is a fundamental mechanism leading to the destruction of neurons in neurodegenerative conditions such as Alzheimer's disease, multiple sclerosis, Parkinson's disease, and Lou Gehrig's disease. Brain cell apoptosis isn't just limited to these disease processes, though. It's occurring in each of us throughout our lifetimes and is responsible for our general decline in brain function as we age.

Until quite recently, scientists subscribed to the paradigm that all cellular functions, including apoptosis, were directed by the cell's nucleus. But as British biochemist Nick Lane notes in his compelling book, *Power, Sex, and Suicide,* "there has been a change in the emphasis that amounts to a revolution, overturning the nascent paradigm. The paradigm was that the nucleus was the operations [center] of the cell, and controls its fate. In many respects this is of course true, but in the case of apoptosis it is not. Remarkably, cells lacking a nucleus can still commit apoptosis. The radical discovery was that mitochondria control the fate of the cell: they determine whether a cell shall live or die."[41]

Mitochondria then, are much more than simple organelles that turn fuel into energy. They wield the sword of Damocles. And it should come as no surprise that they can be damaged very easily by inflammation—especially the kind that originates from disorderly conduct in the gut's microbial community. The gut, after all, is an origin of inflammation given the complex interplay between its microbial inhabitants and the immune system. So inflammatory processes regulated by gut bacteria and resulting in inflammatory molecules coursing through the bloodstream—reaching cells and tissues—will assault the mitochondria.

Moreover, byproducts of an imbalanced gut community can also inflict direct damage to mitochondria and in turn fuel more inflammation. Studies are currently under way to investigate the link between the human microbiome and mitochondrial diseases, especially those that can be passed on to future generations. Mitochondrial diseases include a group of neurological, muscular, and metabolic disorders caused by dysfunctional mitochondria. Disorders as diverse as diabetes, autism, and Alzheimer's have all been linked to mitochondrial problems. In chapter 5, we'll see how mitochondrial dysfunction in children with autism is providing clues to this condition, as well as to the role that the gut bacteria might have in the development of the brain disorder.

With this understanding of the value of mitochondria, it's exciting to know that new mitochondria grow all the time. Perhaps more importantly, we can make lifestyle changes to increase the growth of mitochondria, a process called mitochondrial biogenesis, and thereby enhance an important part of the human microbiome. Lifestyle factors that stimulate this process include eating a diet that derives more energy or calories from fat than from carbohydrate (a central theme of *Grain Brain*), reducing your caloric intake, and engaging in aerobic exercise. Later on in the book I'll go into greater detail about the things you can do to enhance your mitochondria and, in turn, your entire microbiome.

There is one more attribute of the mitochondrial DNA that, to me, has profound implications. All of the mitochondrial DNA is inherited solely from the female lineage. During reproduction, while the nuclear DNA of the sperm joins with that of the egg, the male's mitochondria are excluded. Think of it. Mitochondria, the source of energy to sustain our lives, are the embodiment of a purely feminine genetic code. This concept has prompted scientists to conceive of a "Mitochondrial Eve," the first human mother from whom all humans have derived some of their mitochondrial DNA. Mitochondrial Eve is thought to have lived some 170,000 years ago in East Africa at a time when *Homo sapiens* was developing as a species separate from other hominids. When you consider the fact that bacteria were the planet's original inhabitants, it's no surprise that by the time humans came along, multicellular organisms had long since forged a symbiotic relationship with many bacteria, some of which eventually landed within our own cells to establish a "third dimension" to our genetic fingerprint.

GAINING CONTROL OF MYSTERIOUS ILLNESSES

Perhaps one of the most extraordinary examples of harnessing the power of the gut bacteria to address inflammatory diseases that impact the brain is seen in a patient such as Carlos.

Carlos, forty-three, came to see me in June 2014. He needed a cane to stand and had episodes of feeling as if his legs wouldn't work and as if he could lose his balance easily. When I asked him about his medical history, he told me about one morning back in 1998 when he woke up feeling "drunk and dizzy." When he went to see a neurologist, an MRI scan of his brain was performed, but the results came back normal. Carlos remained unsteady for the next two weeks and then began to feel better. Two weeks after that, while exercising he felt as if ants were crawling down his back. His vision blurred and, hoping to find another opinion about his symptoms, he went to see a naturopath. That's when he began taking various nutritional supplements, and he felt a little better thereafter.

Three years later he had the sudden onset of "numbness in both legs from the waist down." Again he was given a new round of nutritional supplements and after three more months, he felt somewhat improved. Two years later he had another episode, and this similarly resolved itself with more supplements. In 2010, however, he began noticing a progressive decline in his balance and, despite various nutritional supplements, his deterioration continued — rapidly. By 2014, Carlos went through more tests with a neurologist, including another MRI scan of his brain. And this time, his results revealed aggressive abnormalities, especially in the deep white matter of his brain in both hemispheres and even in the brainstem. These findings, in addition to abnormalities noted in an MRI of his cervical spine, a lumbar puncture, and electrical testing results, all pointed to a diagnosis of multiple sclerosis.

MS is an inflammatory disease characterized by damaged nerves in the brain and spinal cord. The insulating covering of these nerve cells, called the myelin, becomes impaired, and so the nervous system breaks down, leading to a wide range of symptoms — physical, cognitive, and even psychiatric. Scientists have long puzzled over what causes multiple sclerosis, though it's generally thought to result from a glitch in the immune system. We just don't know what triggers this glitch, which leads the body to attack its own nerve cells. And yet epidemiological studies have determined that living in an urban environment is a significant risk factor for having this autoimmune disease — similar to the increased risk for developing Alzheimer's disease in urban, Westernized settings.[42]

Could multiple sclerosis — and many other neurological conditions — be directly related to changes that have occurred in the gut's bacterial community? Over the past several years, I've noticed that MS patients almost always were either born by C-section, not breast-fed, or treated with antibiotics for some illness early in life. (In fact, new research published in 2013 showed that the risk of MS was reduced by 42 percent in people who were breast-fed.[43]) In reviewing Carlos's early life experience, once again I found the same pattern to his history: he'd only been breast-fed for several days.

I explained to Carlos that we now understand more about the role gut bacteria play in the immune system, and that recent animal research clearly had identified changes in gut bacteria as possibly playing an important role in this disease. I then offered a plan of action, telling him that I wanted to start a program of probiotic enemas, a technique I'll describe in chapter 9. He agreed without hesitation, administering probiotic-filled enemas two to three times each week. Two weeks later, I received a phone call from him. He indicated that he was walking more comfortably and had now gone for days without the use of a cane! One month later we spoke on the phone again. He was continuing his probiotic enemas three times weekly and felt that he had "stabilized."

At that point I discussed with him the idea of rebuilding a healthy gut population through a revolutionary new procedure called fecal microbial transplantation, or FMT, and he agreed to do so (much more on this technique later; it's currently not available in the U.S. for treating MS). He chose a clinic in England where the procedure is routinely performed on an array of immune and inflammatory problems. Before he left, I asked Carlos to carefully chronicle his experience in a journal and report back to me.

One month after Carlos returned from England we again spoke on the phone. He reported that after his second treatment with fecal transplantation (he received a total of 10) he noted that his walking was dramatically improved and that the improvements were persisting. He told me, "I am walking so well that other people don't know there is anything wrong."

He was so excited about his improvement that he sent me a video of himself walking unassisted. I was thrilled to see how much he had improved and grateful that he allowed me to use the video in my lectures as well as on my website (www.DrPerlmutter.com), where you can find it today. It really completes a story.

I have been practicing neurology for more than three decades and have never witnessed such a remarkable improvement in my patients with multiple sclerosis as I am seeing today with these revolutionary new techniques. I can assure you that I scour the medical journals every month to learn what is new in the treatment of this devastating condition. It is shocking to me that mainstream neurologists don't utilize this approach, and yet, when you put the pieces together and consider the wealth of data already on file in research labs, it sure makes sense.

It certainly made sense for Carlos, whose life was in a downward spiral until we essentially pushed the reset button on his immune system. For me, these experiences are exhilarating; my training had always led me to believe that managing a disease like multiple sclerosis or even considering the idea of a cure would come from some new pharmaceutical development. And now it's becoming patently clear that what may prove to be the most powerful therapy for this disease will be nonproprietary — no one can own it. It's time for the world at large to be made aware that a different perspective on this disease and other mysterious neurological conditions needs to be adopted and embraced.

With all this in mind, let's get emotional. Let's connect the dots between a moody belly and a moody mind. What you're about to learn will probably upend everything you thought you knew about depression, anxiety, and ADHD. And the ultimate brain maker will come closer into view.

CHAPTER 3

Is Your Belly Depressed?

*Why Angry Guts Make for Moody
and Anxious Minds*

By the time Mary came into my office she'd been taking multiple antidepressants and anti-anxiety drugs for more than a year, to no avail. What motivated her to see me was that she was also suffering from serious lapses in memory that made her wonder if she was experiencing early-onset Alzheimer's disease. I quickly ruled that possibility out once I ordered a few tests to get a sense of her mental performance and asked her a handful of questions about her life and lifestyle.

Was she someone who'd been on antibiotics from time to time? Yes. Did she have a diet high in carbohydrates? Yes (in fact, she was struggling to lose weight on a low-fat diet). And was she taking any other medications? Indeed, she was taking statins for high cholesterol, Nexium for acid-reflux, and a sleep aid for insomnia. That was enough to tell me this woman's microbiome was sick and in need of a rehabilitation program.

Three months later, after a few simple tweaks to her diet — the same ones you'll read about in part III — Mary was weaning herself off all the drugs and felt "like a whole new person." Her sharp, calm mind returned, restful sleep descended on her nightly, and she was no longer considered depressed. She'd even lost the extra weight that had bothered her for the better part of the previous decade. Was her transformation atypical? Far from it. Some of my most remarkable case studies involve people changing their lives and health for the better through simple brain-making edits to their dietary choices. They cut carbs and add healthy fats, especially cholesterol—a key player in brain and psychological health. I've watched this fundamental dietary shift single-handedly extinguish depression and all of its kissing cousins, from chronic anxiety to poor memory and even ADHD. In this chapter, I'm going to explain the connections between mental health and gut function. It turns out that if your belly is in a bad mood, so is your mind.

THE SCOPE OF DEPRESSION

The next time you're at a large-scale event with lots of people, whether you're in an auditorium or a stadium, take a look around and consider this: one in ten of those people is taking a psychiatric drug to treat a mood disorder. For women in their forties and fifties, one in four take an antidepressant.[1] That's right, a quarter of middle-aged women today are taking powerful drugs to remedy symptoms that typically fall under a diagnosis of clinical depression: persistent distress, malaise, anxiety, inner agitation, fatigue, low libido, poor memory, irritability, insomnia, sense of hopelessness, and feeling emotionally flat, overwhelmed, and trapped. At last count, 14 percent of non-Hispanic white men take antidepressants, compared with just 4 percent of non-Hispanic blacks and 3 percent of Mexican Americans. Interestingly, antidepressant use does not vary by income status.[2]

As I mentioned in the introduction, depression is now the leading cause of disability worldwide, impacting more than 350 million people (according to the World Health Organization, depression will displace heart disease in terms of cost of caring for patients by the year 2020).

And here in the U.S., rates continue to climb. Last year, 30 million Americans were prescribed $12 billion worth of antidepressants. That means that we are spending more on antidepressants than the Gross National Product of more than half of the world's countries![3]

Ever since serotonin-specific reuptake inhibitor medications (SSRIs) were approved by the FDA nearly three decades ago, we as a society have come to believe that drugs can improve symptoms of or even "cure" mental illness, particularly depression, anxiety disorders, and panic attacks, which together are the top targets of medication in the U.S. Such drug use has increased a whopping 400 percent over the past two decades. By 2005, antidepressants had become the #1 prescribed drug class in the country.[4]

But these medications do not treat depression. Whether it's Prozac, Cymbalta, Zoloft, Elavil, Lexapro, Wellbutrin, or any of the other commonly prescribed antidepressants, these medicines simply treat symptoms, and only minimally so. Drugs for depression are aggressively marketed and prescribed in this country; look no further than the direct-to-consumer advertisements that dominate in broadcast media. The same is true of ADHD drugs: 85 percent of drugs to treat ADHD are used in the U.S. Although children are still the primary users of these drugs, the number of adults using them has been increasing at a much faster pace lately. The percentage of kids taking them increased 18 percent between 2008 and 2012, but during that same time period the percentage of privately insured adults who take them skyrocketed 53 percent.[5] I am saddened by the fact that the billion-dollar psychotropic pharmaceutical industry is predicated on the idea that people will take a pill to treat symptoms, while the underlying disorder is ignored. So there's never any real focus on actually curing or even improving the root cause of the illness, let alone getting people off the medication.

From a business perspective, this certainly makes sense as it generates repeat, lifetime customers. And we Americans are lulled into believing that this is what we should expect. As a physician, I read medical journals daily that are peppered with ads for antidepressants. It's no wonder that in this age of rationing healthcare, and given the demands placed upon doctors to see as many patients as possible, the quick-fix mentality and the prescription pad have become the norm. This approach is categorically wrong and fraught with potentially devastating consequences. What's also disturbing is the fact that most prescriptions for antidepressants are written by primary-care physicians — not mental health professionals.

We need to focus on understanding the causes of mental illness, so that we can find real treatments and cures that don't involve potentially dangerous drugs with serious side effects. And you know where I'm going with this; it's now become clear that what's going on in the gut determines, to some degree, what happens in the brain. The research exploring the connection between the gut and psychiatric issues is now narrowing in on the microbiome. A number of mechanisms — most of which are now familiar to you — are at play, including the direct effects of gut bacteria on the intestinal barrier, and their effects on the production of neurotransmitters that impact mental wellness.

All of the antidepressant medications currently on the market are designed to artificially alter neurotransmitter activity in the brain. Yet, when we consider the fact that these same chemicals found in the brain are also produced in the gut, and that their availability to the brain is largely governed by the activity of gut bacteria, we are forced to realize that ground zero for all things mood-related is the gut.

As a neurologist, for example, I find it intriguing to note that today's antidepressants purportedly work by increasing the availability of the neurotransmitter serotonin,[6] and yet the precursor for serotonin — tryptophan — is tightly regulated by the gut bacteria. In fact, a particular bacterium, *Bifidobacterium infantis*, does a great job of making tryptophan available.[7]

The previous chapter gave you a bird's-eye view of the power of the microbiome through the lens of inflammation. If you were to ask someone on the street about depression, you'd be likely to hear something along the lines of "It's a chemical imbalance in the brain." Well, I'm here to tell you that that would be incorrect. Two decades of scientific literature highlight the role of inflammation in mental illness, from depression to schizophrenia. The field of psychiatry has known about the role of the immune system in the onset of depression for the better part of the last century. But only recently have we begun to understand the connection, thanks to better technology and longitudinal studies. Not only do our gut's microbes control the production of inflammatory chemicals in the body that factor into mental health, but they control our ability to absorb certain nutrients—such as omega-3 fats—and manufacture vitamins key to mental health. Let's take a tour of the latest science.

DEPRESSION IS AN INFLAMMATORY DISEASE

The connection between depression and the gut is not new information.[8] In the early part of the 20th century, scientists and clinicians were deeply involved in this research, thinking that toxic chemicals being manufactured in the gut could affect mood and brain function. This process even had a name: "auto intoxication." More than eighty years ago a team of scientists wrote: "It is far from our mind to conceive that all mental conditions have the same etiological factor, but we feel justified in recognizing the existence of cases of mental disorders which have as a basic etiological factor a toxic condition arising in the gastrointestinal tract."[9]

Unfortunately, studying the gut and dietary patterns began to be viewed as "unscientific." By mid-century the idea that the gut's contents could affect mental health had rapidly vanished, replaced by the notion that depression and anxiety were important factors in influencing the gut—not the other way around. As the pharmaceutical industry exploded, these prescient researchers were disregarded. How incredible that more than eighty years later we have come full circle.

Today, much of the focus is on studies that show a link between gut dysfunction and the brain, and, more specifically, the link between the presence of inflammatory markers in the blood (indicating that the body's immune system is on high alert) and risk for depression. Higher levels of inflammation dramatically increase the risk of developing depression.[10] And the higher the levels of inflammatory markers, the worse the depression.[11] This places depression right in line with other inflammatory disorders such as Parkinson's disease, multiple sclerosis, and Alzheimer's disease.

Depression can no longer be viewed as a disorder rooted solely in the brain. Some of the studies have been downright eye-opening. For example, when scientists give healthy people with no signs of depression an infusion of a substance to trigger inflammation (more on this shortly), classic depressive symptoms develop almost instantly.[12] Similarly, it's been shown that when people are given interferon for the treatment of hepatitis C, which increases inflammatory cytokines, a quarter of those individuals develop major depression.[13] Interferons are a group of naturally occurring proteins that form an integral part of the immune system, but they can be made and given as a drug to treat certain viral infections.

What's even more compelling is new research demonstrating that antidepressant medications may work in some people by virtue of their ability to decrease inflammatory chemicals.[14] Put another way, the actual mechanism for modern antidepressants may have nothing at all to do with their effect on serotonin and everything to do with decreasing inflammation. Unfortunately, this doesn't mean that antidepressants are always effective. Even if they can alleviate symptoms through their anti-inflammatory effects (and/or placebo effects), they aren't getting to the source of the problem and putting out the fire. They are, in a sense, poorly constructed Band-Aids over cuts that won't heal.

When I think about our soaring rates of depression, I wonder about the impact of our sedentary lifestyles and diets that are loaded with pro-inflammatory sugars, too many pro-inflammatory omega-6 fats, and too few anti-inflammatory omega-3 fats. We know, for example, that the typical Western diet — high in refined carbs and factory fats — is associated with higher levels of C-reactive protein, a popular marker of inflammation.[15] A diet filled with foods that are high on the glycemic index is also associated with higher levels of C-reactive protein.[16] The glycemic index is a scale of 0 to 100, with higher values indicating foods that cause the fastest and most persistent elevations in blood sugar. Pure glucose, which has a GI of 100, provides the reference point. Foods high on the glycemic index notoriously increase inflammation.

High blood sugar, in fact, is one of the biggest risk factors for depression, just as it is for Alzheimer's.[17] Although we used to think that diabetes and depression were two distinct disorders, thinking on this is changing. A large landmark study spanning 10 years and following more than 65,000 women, published in 2010 in the *Archives of Internal Medicine,* shone a blinding light on the relationship: women with diabetes were nearly 30 percent more likely to develop depression.[18] This was true even after the researchers took into account other depression risk factors, such as weight and lack of physical exercise. And those women who took insulin for their diabetes were 53 percent more likely to develop depression. I think it's telling that as we've watched diabetes rates soar in the past twenty years, we've seen a similar increase in rates of depression. It should come as no surprise that obesity is also associated with increased inflammatory markers. Obesity is correlated with a 55 percent increased risk of depression, while depression is associated with a 58 percent increased risk of developing obesity.[19]

So powerful is the relationship between depression and inflammation that researchers are now exploring the use of immune-altering medications to treat depression. But where is this inflammation coming from? To quote one team of Belgian researchers: "There is now evidence that major depression (MDD) is accompanied by an activation of the inflammatory response system and that pro-inflammatory cytokines and lipopolysaccharide (LPS) may induce depressive symptoms."[20] In case you missed the trigger word, it's LPS—the incendiary device that I introduced in the previous chapter. In 2008, these researchers documented a significant increase in the level of antibodies against LPS in the blood of individuals with major depression. (Interestingly, the authors also commented on the fact that major depression is often accompanied by gastrointestinal symptoms. One explanation might be the fallout from a disrupted gut community.) Their findings were so incontrovertible that the authors emphatically recommended that patients suffering from major depression should be checked for leaky gut by measuring these antibodies, and subsequently treated for this problem.

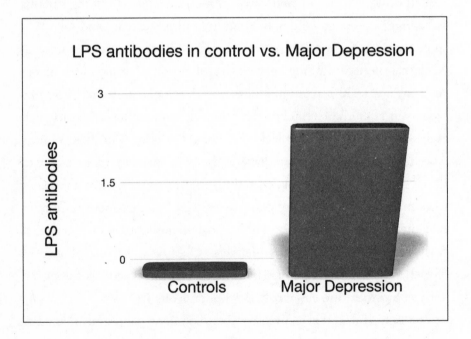

Researchers around the world are finally looking at LPS and its role in depression.[21] As we've discussed, inflammatory markers correlate with depression, and LPS increases the production of these inflammatory chemicals. And here's where it gets really compelling: not only does

LPS make the gut more permeable, but it can cross the blood-brain barrier and allow pro-inflammatory chemicals to bombard the brain. This is true for dementia, too, and as the authors of one 2013 study stated, "Among those with depression, the subsequent risk of dementia or mild cognitive impairment is up to twofold higher and researchers continue to evaluate low-grade inflammation as a primary driver of cognitive decline."[22]

To my mind, studies like this represent a "smoking gun." The movement of LPS through the gut wall lights a fire in the body and brain, which can result in depression and, later on, dementia. Depression is in fact far more common in people with other inflammatory and auto-immune issues like irritable bowel syndrome, chronic fatigue syndrome, fibromyalgia, insulin resistance, and obesity. All of these conditions are characterized by higher levels of both inflammation and intestinal permeability, and this is why we must focus on the gut.

Plenty of studies have begun to look at how our diet may be responsible for increased gut permeability as well as loss of bacterial diversity. And connections are finally being made between diet and risk for depression. The science is showing that people who stick to a Mediterranean-type diet, rich in healthy, anti-inflammatory fats and proteins, enjoy significantly lower rates of depression.[23] Conversely, a diet high in carbs and sugar sets up an "inflammatory microbiome." We can even examine the effects of specific ingredients on the body's inflammatory pathways; for example, fructose has been shown to increase circulating LPS by 40 percent.[24] But this can be reversed back to normal when fructose is removed or severely restricted in the diet and the balance of gut microbes is shifted. High-fructose corn syrup now represents 42 percent of all caloric sweeteners, which could be a factor in our soaring rates of depression and even dementia. Later on, we'll see what kinds of ingredients—cocoa, coffee, and curcumin (turmeric), for example—can have the opposite effect of lowering the risk of depression by helping balance the microbiome.

AUTOIMMUNE DISEASE, INFECTION, AND DEPRESSION

I've already hinted at a connection between autoimmune disease and risk for depression. In 2013, a collaborative team of researchers from various institutions in Denmark and Johns Hopkins School of Public Health reported on a large group of people who were followed between 1945 and 1996.[25] Of the 3.56 million individuals tracked during that time period, 91,637 were hospitalized because of mood disorders. These researchers performed a few elegant calculations and managed to figure out that being hospitalized because of an autoimmune disease increased the risk of being hospitalized for a mood disorder by 45 percent. Moreover, any history of being in the hospital for an infection increased the risk of getting diagnosed with a mood disorder later on by a whopping 62 percent. And for those who experienced both an autoimmune disease and infection, their risk for a mood disorder more than doubled.

Although we tend to isolate these matters in our minds, not considering a link between, say, having influenza as a young adult and developing depression later in life, research like this further demonstrates the tie that binds: inflammation. In the case of an infection, the immune system fans the flames as it tries to fight the infection. If antibiotics come into the picture, they will degrade the microbiome and further facilitate the inflammatory process. Drugs to treat autoimmune disease, such as steroids, can also tinker with the balance of gut bacteria as well as change the functionality of the immune system.

The authors of the study, which was published in *JAMA Psychiatry*, a specialty journal from the American Medical Association, concluded that autoimmune diseases and infections are risk factors for developing mood disorders. Indeed, your medical history—and I mean across your whole life span—factors into whether or not you'll be diagnosed with a psychiatric condition today or in the future. A handful of studies, for example, have suggested that a history of not being breast-fed early in life may be associated with a higher risk of major depression later in life. In one such study of 52 adults with a diagnosis of major depression and 106 healthy controls who never suffered depression, researchers found that 72 percent of the people who had never reported depression were breast-fed, whereas only 46 percent of the patients with depression had been breast-fed.[26]

CHANGE YOUR GUT, CHANGE YOUR MOOD

Although the studies showing the gut-brain axis and the relationship between the intestinal microbiome and mental health do go back many years, it seems that only recently have scientists really begun to dig deep into studying this connection and how one can manipulate gut bacteria to improve mental health. In 2011, a study from McMaster University in Ontario, Canada, was among the first to really show that the gut itself can communicate with the brain and influence behavior.[27] In their investigation, the researchers compared the behaviors of mice whose guts had been stripped of microbes and behaviors of normal mice. The bacteria-free mice not only displayed more risk-taking, but they also had higher levels of the stress hormone cortisol and reduced levels of the brain chemical BDNF. Lower levels of BDNF have long been associated with human anxiety and depression.

Further research from this same group has further confirmed such findings. In another study, this one published in *Gastroenterology*, the researchers showed that they could switch a mouse's gut bacteria with that of another and significantly alter behavior.[28] They transplanted microbes from a timid group of mice into the guts of risk-taking mice and watched their personalities change. The shy mice became outgoing; the brazen mice became apprehensive. In the words of the study's lead author, Jane Foster: "It's good evidence that the microbiota houses these behaviors."[29]

A team of UCLA researchers conducted a nifty little experiment published in 2013, also in the journal *Gastroenterology*, that produced some of the first evidence that friendly bacteria consumed from food can affect brain function in humans.[30] Although it was a small study, it nonetheless got people in the medical community talking, because it basically showed how small changes in the gut bacteria affect how a person perceives the world.

Thirty-six women were split into three groups: Group 1 consumed, twice daily for four weeks, a yogurt mixture containing several probiotics; Group 2 ate a dairy product that looked and tasted like yogurt but didn't have any probiotics; and Group 3 ate no specific product at all. At the beginning of the study, each subject underwent a functional MRI (fMRI) scan of the brain that was repeated after four weeks. Rather than looking at the structures of the brain, fMRI evaluates brain activity so that researchers can determine which areas of the brain are active and how active they are at any particular time. When we neurologists observe such activity, we technically call it "excitability"—how the brain responds to stimuli or changes in the environment. At the four-week point, participants were shown images designed to induce an emotional response. Specifically, they viewed a series of pictures of angry or frightened people and matched them to other faces showing the same emotions.

What the scientists found was truly remarkable. The women who ate the yogurt that contained the probiotics showed decreased activity in both the insula and the somatosensory cortex during the emotional reactivity task. The insula is the part of the brain that processes and integrates internal body sensations, like those from the gut. These women also had less activity, or excitability, in the brain's widespread network related to emotion, cognition, and sensory processing. The women in the other two groups, on the other hand, exhibited stable or increased activity in this network, indicating that they were emotionally impacted and disturbed by the images. What's more, when the researchers scanned subjects' brains without engaging them in the emotional reactivity task, the women consuming probiotics displayed greater connectivity between a key brainstem region and areas of the prefrontal cortex associated with cognition. But the women who didn't eat any product showed greater connectivity to regions of the brain associated with emotion and sensation. The group consuming the non-probiotic dairy product showed results in between.

The study's senior author, Dr. Emeran Mayer, a professor of medicine, physiology, and psychiatry, stated the implications of the findings perfectly for UCLA's press release: "The knowledge that signals are sent from the intestine to the brain and that they can be modulated by a dietary change is likely to lead to an expansion of research aimed at finding new strategies to prevent or treat digestive, mental and neurological disorders."[31] He then went on to articulate the heart of his conclusions: "There are studies showing that what we eat can alter the composition and products of the gut flora—in particular, that people with high-vegetable, fiber-based diets have a different composition of their microbiota, or gut environment, than people who eat the more typical Western diet that is high in fat and carbohydrates...Now we know that this has an effect not only on the metabolism but also affects brain function." I spoke with Dr. Mayer about his research at a conference recently, complimenting him on his findings. He very humbly responded that yes, the results were exciting, but more research needs to be done.

The fact that changes in our gut affect our brain's response to negativity or emotionally stirring images is just mind-boggling. But it's also empowering. It means that what we put in our mouths and how we feed our gut bacteria do indeed affect our brain's functionality.

IT WORKS BOTH WAYS

It's important to bear in mind that while we've been exploring the relationship of the gut to the brain, a relatively new concept in medicine, we can't forget that the brain can wield its own sword over the gut as well.[32] This can create a vicious cycle, whereby psychological stress and anxiety can actually increase gut permeability and change the complexion of the gut bacteria, leading to increased leakiness of the gut and further inflammation. Much research has been conducted recently that looks at the hypothalamic-pituitary-adrenal axis (HPA axis). Broadly speaking, the HPA axis stimulates the adrenal glands during times of stress to create the chemical cortisol. Cortisol is the body's key stress response hormone. It's made by the adrenals, which sit atop the kidneys, and it serves to help us in times of fight or flight—the instinctive physiological response to a threatening situation, which prepares us to either run away or combat the threat. But you can get too much of a good thing: Higher levels of cortisol correlate with a variety of issues, including depression and Alzheimer's disease.

Elevated cortisol also has some damaging effects on the gut. First, it changes the mix of gut bacteria. Second, it increases permeability of the gut lining by triggering the release of chemicals from cells; multiple studies have shown that these chemicals, which include TNF-α, directly assault the gut lining.[33] And third, cortisol enhances production of inflammatory chemicals coming from immune cells. These cytokines ramp up inflammation in the gut, leading to further permeability, and also directly and negatively stimulate the brain, making it more susceptible to mood disorders.

Although anecdotal evidence alone will tell you that being stressed out can cause an upset stomach and even be associated with intestinal diseases, we now have the scientific evidence to explain how this happens. The latest research indicates that chronic stress may be more harmful than acute stress in terms of gut permeability and inflammation. It also tells us that gut bacteria control, to a large extent, the body's stress response. In one particularly revealing study published in 2004 in the *Journal of Physiology*, Japanese researchers documented the effects of stress on mice that lacked a microbiome ("germ-free mice").[34] The mice overreacted, as it were, to stress. They had an exaggerated HPA response, meaning an outflow of more damaging cortisol. The good news is that this state could be reversed just by giving them the probiotic *Bifidobacterium infantis*. I marvel at the thought that my gut's bugs, rather than my brain, can control my response to stress.

GUT BACTERIA AND A GOOD NIGHT'S SLEEP

The stress hormone cortisol is uniquely tied to our circadian rhythm — the ebb and flow of hormones through the 24-hour day that factors into our biology and whether or not we're feeling alert or tired. Insomnia is a common symptom in mood-related disorders, and it's now known to be linked to the microbiome. New research is showing that many cytokines such as certain interleukins and TNF-α are important for inducing sleep, particularly deep, non-REM sleep, the most restorative kind. And it's gut bacteria that stimulate production of these chemicals in concert with cortisol levels.[35]

Cortisol levels are supposed to be naturally lowest at night, beginning to rise in the early morning hours. Cytokines essentially have circadian cycles dictated by gut bacteria. When cortisol levels go up in the morning, the gut bacteria inhibit production of cytokines, and this shift defines the transition between non-REM and REM sleep. Hence, disruption of the gut bacteria can have significant negative effects on sleep and circadian rhythms. Balance the gut, break through the insomnia.

ANXIOUS BUGS

With all this in mind, let's briefly turn our attention to anxiety, a relative of depression. The two often go hand in hand—someone with chronic anxiety can be diagnosed as depressed and recommended to take antidepressants alongside anti-anxiety medications. It's common to suffer from both anxiety and depression at the same time, and sometimes persistent anxiety is what leads to depressive symptoms due to its impact on one's life. The chief difference between the two disorders, however, is that anxiety is characterized by fear and apprehension, nervous thoughts, and exaggerated worries about the future. Depression, on the other hand, doesn't entail such fears and rather revolves around a sense of hopelessness. So, rather than thinking "the sky is *going* to fall," people with depression feel that the sky has already fallen, that life is bad and nothing can go right.

Nonetheless, anxiety and depression are often talked about in the same conversation because they are related psychologically (i.e., both involve a lot of negative thinking) and they do have many physical symptoms in common (e.g., headaches, pain, nausea, GI problems). There are many types of anxiety disorders, just as there is a wide spectrum of depression, but the two conditions have a lot in common in terms of the state of the gut bacteria. As with depression, anxiety is strongly related to a disruption of the gut microbiota. Numerous studies have found the same kinds of features in people with anxiety disorder as in those with depression: higher levels of inflammation in the gut, higher levels of systemic inflammation, lower levels of the brain's growth hormone BDNF (especially in the hippocampus), higher levels of cortisol and an over-reactive stress response, and increased permeability of the gut.[36, 37, 38, 39] Sound familiar?

It's natural to feel anxious and even depressed on occasion, but when these emotions are unrelenting and cause such distress that they interfere with quality of life, they become matters of mental illness. Anxiety disorders affect about 40 million American adults in any given year. These include panic disorder, obsessive-compulsive disorder, social phobia, and generalized anxiety disorder.[40] And while the research is still in its infancy, it's becoming clear that anxiety disorders, as well as depression, are caused by a combination of factors that most definitely include the state and function of the gut and its inhabitants.

Although the final straw in triggering an anxiety disorder may very well be misfires in those parts of the brain that control fear and other emotions, we can't negate the fact that such neural transmissions partly depend on the health of the microbiome. When the balance of gut bacteria isn't right, other biological pathways—be they hormonal, immunological, or neuronal—aren't right, either. And the brain's processing centers, such as those that handle emotions, can be mightily affected. In my own experience, I've found that patients report never feeling anxious or depressed until they started having problems with their guts. Coincidence? I think not. Thankfully, studies are finally starting to emerge that show the connection.

In a 2011 study published in the *Proceedings of the National Academy of Sciences*, mice fed probiotics had significantly lower levels of the stress hormone corticosterone than mice fed plain broth. The bacteria-fed mice also exhibited much less behavior linked with stress, anxiety, and depression than mice fed plain broth.[41] What's also interesting is that both animal and human studies have shown that certain probiotics, ones I describe in chapter 10, can alleviate anxiety by rebalancing the microbiome.[42] In a recent study, for example, Oxford University neurobiologists found that giving people prebiotics—"food" for good bacteria—resulted in positive psychological effects.[43] Forty-five healthy adults between the ages of eighteen and forty-five took either a prebiotic or placebo every day for three weeks. The participants were then tested so the researchers could gauge their processing of emotional information. The underlying theory was that if you're anxious to begin with, you'll be more reactive to negativity, such as emotionally charged images or words.

Indeed, the Oxford researchers documented that, as compared to the placebo group, the individuals who'd taken the prebiotic paid more attention to positive information and less attention to negative information. This effect, which has been observed among individuals on antidepressants or anti-anxiety medication, suggested that the prebiotic group had less anxiety when confronted with the negative stimuli. Interestingly, the researchers also discovered that the people who took the prebiotics had lower levels of cortisol, as measured through their saliva in the morning when cortisol is supposed to be highest. This study wasn't too dissimilar from the UCLA one using a fermented milk product, but it's important in that it adds to the volume of human studies showing a relationship between gut bacteria and mental health, especially with regard to anxiety.

I must bring in one more important nugget of data here that really helps define what's going on in the body of an anxious (and probably depressed) person. As you'll recall, serotonin is an important neurotransmitter, one that's often linked to feelings of well-being. It's synthesized from the amino acid tryptophan, but when tryptophan is degraded in the body by certain enzymes, it becomes unavailable for the production of serotonin. One of the byproducts of broken-down tryptophan is kynurenine, so high levels of kynurenine are a good indicator of low tryptophan levels.

Elevated levels of kynurenine are routinely documented not only in patients with depression and anxiety but also Alzheimer's disease, cardiovascular disease, and even in people with tic disorders. In the future, my hope is that we begin to treat these ailments with probiotics, because it's already known, for example, that the probiotic I just mentioned, *Bifidobacterium infantis* — the same one shown to calm the stress response — is associated with lower levels of kynurenine.[44] This means that more tryptophan is available to be used for the production of serotonin, which is key to staving off not just depression but anxiety as well.

Take Martina, a 56-year-old woman who came to see me for anxiety and depression. Her story helps illustrate the connection between mental health and the microbiome.

Martina was fed up with taking medicines that weren't working for ten years, but she was afraid to quit. At the time she was taking an antidepressant, as well as a non-steroid anti-inflammatory for chronic pain in her arms and legs that had previously been diagnosed as fibromyalgia. In reviewing her history, I noted that she began to have issues with depression in her early 20s but hadn't started medication until her mid-40s. She had been born naturally but not breast-fed. She had been on multiple courses of antibiotics as a child for throat infections that culminated in a tonsillectomy. During her teenage years she had been placed on the antibiotic tetracycline for eighteen months because of acne. Bowel movements had always been a problem; Martina said she'd suffered from either chronic constipation or diarrhea for "as long as I can remember."

The first thing I did was order some laboratory studies. That's when I found out that she was significantly sensitive to gluten. Her vitamin D level was low, and her LPS level, a marker of gut permeability and inflammation, was sky-high.

I explained that our main mission moving forward was to restore the health of her gut. I recommended a gluten-free diet and an aggressive oral probiotic program, along with prebiotic foods and vitamin D supplementation. I made several other lifestyle-based suggestions, including regular aerobic exercise and more hours of sleep.

I saw Martina six weeks later and, even before our conversation began, it was clear that she had been transformed. She looked radiant. In our clinic we photograph all of our patients at the initial examination. I took another picture now and we looked at them side by side. It was an outstanding comparison (go to www.DrPerlmutter.com to see for yourself).

Though I hadn't recommended it, she had stopped her antidepressant four weeks prior to this appointment and was now off all medications. "I feel like the fog has finally lifted," she reported. And her chronic anxiety had vanished. She was sleeping well, enjoying her exercise, and, for the first time in decades, having regular bowel movements. I asked her about her fibromyalgia pain and she said that she hadn't mentioned it as she had forgotten all about it.

YOUNG, DISTRACTED, AND DRUGGED

Perhaps there's no better way to understand the relationship between a moody belly and an unstable mind than to consider one particular group of people: children with ADHD. Although adults are routinely diagnosed with ADHD, it is the children who in my opinion are in danger because their brains are still very much under construction. While ADHD and depression are often spoken about separately, they have a lot in common. After all, some of their symptoms are the same, and they both have the same underlying mechanism: rampant inflammation.[45] Moreover, both are treated with powerful, mind-altering drugs rather than through diet. In fact, in some cases, ADHD is treated with antidepressants.

Today more than 11 percent of children aged four to seventeen are diagnosed as having ADHD, and a staggering two-thirds of these kids are medicated. On the Centers for Disease Control and Prevention's website, the homepage for ADHD includes facts about symptoms and diagnosis, then moves right to treatment options, none of which include a dietary protocol. There is not a single mention of prevention.

American children are not genetically different to any significant degree from children of other nations where ADHD is rarely seen (as mentioned, the vast majority of ADHD medications used in the world are used right here in the U.S., and that is something we don't need to be proud of). No one is asking the obvious, billion-dollar question: why are children in Western cultures having such issues as attention deficit, learning disabilities, and impulsivity control problems? Obviously what's going on here is something environmental. Something has changed, something modifiable. Frightening new data shows that more than 10,000 American toddlers (two- and three-year-olds) are now being medicated for ADHD.[46] Treating children at this age with pharmaceuticals is totally outside of established pediatric guidelines. There is virtually no data explaining what these potent drugs do to the developing brain. Even more disturbing is the fact that children on Medicaid are more likely to be placed on stimulating drugs like Ritalin and Adderall than kids in middle- and upper-class families.[47] That is to say, lower-income children are far more likely to be treated with drugs.

Although concerns over the use of these drugs have prompted the popularity of so-called "non-stimulant" approaches to the treatment of ADHD, alternative drugs are proving no less problematic. Drugs like ato-moxetine (Strattera) come with their own basket of unpleasant side effects (drowsiness, low energy, loss of appetite, nausea, vomiting, stom-ach cramps, trouble sleeping, dry mouth, and so on). And beyond side effects, research shows that this drug actually stimulates the expression of 114 genes while silencing 11 others.[48] Yet doctors continue to write pre-scriptions. In the words of one team of researchers whose study high-lighted these genetic changes, "Little is known about the molecular basis for its therapeutic effect."[49]

I spend a lot of time in my clinical practice treating children with ADHD. Part of my clinical exam involves taking a medical history. Pre-dictably, parents of children with ADHD often tell me that their child had frequent ear infections for which antibiotics were prescribed. Some of these children had their tonsils removed, and many were not breast-fed for long, if at all. Many of them were born by cesarean section.

In 2000, a study came out in the *American Journal of Clinical Nutrition* in which Purdue University's Dr. Laura J. Stevens revealed that children who were breast-fed were far less likely to be diagnosed with ADHD; she also noted a relationship between how long a mother breast-fed and the risk of the child developing ADHD.[50] Even more enlightening was her finding that having a lot of ear infections and exposure to antibiotics was highly associated with increased risk for ADHD. In another prominent study I highlighted in chapter 1, children who were born by C-section had triple the risk of ADHD. In other words, ADHD doesn't just happen at random.[51]

All of these correlations point to changes in gut bacteria. As you know, method of birth and breastfeeding are critical in establishing the right balance of organisms in the gut, which then goes on to create a stable environment for the body's appropriate response to immune challenges. Antibiotics change the complexion of gut bacteria, thereby compromising the intestinal wall and changing the brain's response to what goes on in the gut. This can mean changing levels of important neurotransmitters and increasing the production of inflammatory chemicals that are irritating to the brain and can compromise brain function. The production of essential vitamins important for brain function is also disrupted. The cumulative impact of all these events is inflammation, which is detrimental to the brain both in the short- and long-term. In the case of ADHD, individuals with genetic predispositions to the disorder and who suffer from chronic inflammation are at a high risk for developing the condition. It's no surprise to me that the increase in cases of ADHD has paralleled the rise in childhood obesity, another inflammatory condition linked to the gut bacteria that we'll explore in chapter 4.

I also am no longer taken aback by how often my ADHD patients have digestive complaints. Chronic constipation is a given in most cases, even among those not taking a stimulant, which can also cause constipation. But I'm not the only one who's made this observation. In a recent publication in the journal *Pediatrics*, researchers evaluated a group of 742,939 children, 32,773 of whom (4.4 percent) had ADHD.[52] The prevalence of constipation was almost threefold higher in the kids with ADHD. Fecal incontinence (loss of bowel control) was 67 percent higher in the ADHD group. And there was no difference in these rates whether the children were taking medication for ADHD or not.

This kind of large-scale data makes it clear that something is going on in the digestive systems of these children, and that it relates directly to brain function. Moreover, German researchers recently revealed a high prevalence of gluten sensitivity in children with ADHD. The researchers placed those individuals found to be gluten-sensitive on a gluten-free diet and reported that, "after initiation of the gluten-free diet, patients or their parents reported a significant improvement in their behavior and functioning compared to the before period."[53] The authors went on to recommend testing for gluten sensitivity as part of the evaluation process for ADHD. They also stated that ADHD should not be viewed as a distinct disorder, but rather as a *symptom* of various other issues. I couldn't agree more. ADHD is simply a manifestation of inflammation gone awry due to triggers like gluten and the downstream effects of a sick microbiome.

In fact, dietary factors alone have also been implicated in the development of ADHD. Aside from the effects we already know of diet on the microbiome, researchers have shown that many children's behavioral challenges can be remedied effectively with dietary changes. According to a study published in the *Lancet* in 2011, researchers documented a staggering improvement of symptoms of ADHD through a restricted diet.[54] Although this wasn't the first time that diet has been incriminated in the development of (and sustainment of) ADHD, it was the first to really shine a light on impact of diet on a brain disorder like ADHD. The researchers went so far as to suggest that more than half of children diagnosed with ADHD may actually be experiencing a hypersensitivity to food—foods like dairy, wheat, and processed products with artificial ingredients and food colorings. Although this study did have its critics and more studies are needed, it nonetheless opened the conversation up to factoring in dietary influences on ADHD. Such a study once again reiterates the possibility that a behavioral disorder like ADHD originates from external factors (e.g., diet)—and can be treated through changes to one's environment. This includes changes to the microbiome, for dietary shifts result in shifts in the composition of gut bacteria, which in turn may impact behavior.

Let me share one more piece of the puzzle that ties everything back to the gut. It involves GABA, the important neurotransmitter I've discussed before. This chemical is largely deficient in the brains of ADHD children. An ingenious study carried out by Dr. Richard Edden, associate professor of radiology at Johns Hopkins University School of Medicine, used a sophisticated technology called magnetic resonance spectroscopy that, figuratively speaking, opens a window into the brain, allowing scientists to measure various chemicals in living people.[55] The researchers applied this technology to a group of children ranging in age from eight to twelve years and noted a significant difference in brain concentrations of GABA in the two groups. The ADHD group had much lower levels of GABA compared to the control group. They concluded that ADHD may well be the result of a GABA deficiency.

What's triggering this lack of GABA, and how we can increase GABA in the brains of these kids? GABA is manufactured in the body from the amino acid glutamine. But the conversion of glutamine to GABA requires the presence of what are called cofactors, chemicals necessary for a specific chemical reaction to take place. Specifically, the conversion demands both zinc and vitamin B6—two ingredients that must come from food. GABA can then be created by specific varieties of gut bacteria using these cofactors. Now scientists are trying to figure out which strains are involved in GABA's production. Researchers reporting in the *Journal of Applied Microbiology* have so far discovered that specific types of *Lactobacillus* and *Bifidobacterium* produce GABA in abundance.[56] Moreover, studies using these bacteria in probiotic form have already shown promise in reducing anxiety.[57, 58]

A lot of research is being conducted now on GABA and its relationship to specific components of ADHD-like impulsivity.[59] Researchers are also exploring GABA and its potential connection to another brain disorder: Tourette syndrome.[60] The overriding consensus about why a lack of GABA can be so impactful in the brain seems to be that it's an inhibitory neurotransmitter—it decreases a neuron's electrical charge, thereby making it less likely to excite nearby neurons. Deficiencies in GABA activity would mean that areas of the brain would be put into overdrive, and this would certainly fit with what we observe in kids with the excessive motor activity characteristic of Tourette syndrome as well as loss of impulse control. (More on Tourette syndrome in chapter 9.)

As I've said, we've got to get away from the notion that we can fix our brain-related issues with pharmaceutical interventions that affect symptoms but ignore the underlying cause—especially when it comes to children. Imagine if we could treat children with ADHD by using healthy diet, probiotics, and other nutritional supplements instead of Ritalin. One promising study on this was published back in 2003—five years before the Human Microbiome Project commenced. The researchers evaluated twenty children with ADHD.[61] Half of the children received Ritalin while the other half received probiotics like *Lactobacillus acidophilus* and nutritional supplements including essential fatty acids.

To the researchers' astonishment, the probiotics and supplements provided the same outcome as Ritalin. These authors noted that "essential lipids" repairing the cells lining the gut, along with "re-inoculation of friendly flora and the administration of probiotics," might well explain the positive outcome in these children. This information published over a decade ago offers an alternative to the use of potentially dangerous drugs. Although it was a small study and more research in this realm is needed, I expect many more studies to emerge, adding to the evidence that there's a strong connection between ADHD and the balance of healthy gut bacteria.[62] We already have thirty-five years of research examining the link between dietary sensitivities and symptoms of ADHD.[63] Now we just have to further document the role of the gut bacteria in this big picture.

Earlier I mentioned how the rise in ADHD has mirrored the upward spiral in childhood obesity. Over the past two decades, we've watched the number of incidences of both conditions soar to unprecedented heights. And, as I've shown, they most definitely share ties with the microbiome. Now that you've gotten a sense of how gut bacteria play into mood and anxiety disorders, it's time to turn to the other elephant in the room. Is our microbiome rather than our penchant for cake and Coke responsible for the obesity epidemic, including the one affecting our children? Let's go there next.

CHAPTER 4

How Your Intestinal Flora Can Make You Fat and Brainsick

The Surprising Links Between Your Gut's Bacteria and Appetite, Obesity, and the Brain

YOU KNOW HOW DREADFUL THE obesity epidemic is because your eyes gloss over the headlines all the time. The numbers are so huge now that they really do cause one to want to brush them aside. Worldwide, the number of overweight and obese people increased from 857 million in 1982 to 2.1 billion in 2013, a growth of more than 145 percent.[1] Another way of grasping the enormity of this problem is to consider that in 1990 less than 15 percent of the U.S. population was obese in most states. By 2010, 36 states had obesity rates of 25 percent or higher, and 12 of those states had obesity rates of 30 percent or higher. Nationwide today, approximately two out of three adults are overweight or obese.[2] Current standards say that someone with a body mass index (BMI, a measure of weight relative to a person's height) of 25 to 29.9 is "overweight"; "obese" refers to those with a BMI of 30 or higher.

Obesity affects slightly more women than men, and 26 percent of children in the U.S. are now classified as obese. Obesity costs us $147 billion annually to treat. Globally, 3.4 million people die each year from causes related to being overweight or obese.[3] And health consequences go far beyond the psychological burden of dealing with the condition. In addition to taking an emotional toll on the individual, who perceives prejudice and discrimination due to their obesity and faces the stigma of obesity every day, being overweight or obese is associated with cardiovascular disease, cancer, diabetes, osteoarthritis, chronic kidney disease, and neurodegenerative ailments, including Alzheimer's disease. Unfortunately, the effects of obesity on the brain are often not part of the conversation. But they should be. We now have unmistakable and irrefutable scientific evidence that being overweight or obese significantly increases the chances of cognitive decline, loss of brain tissue, and the full array of various brain diseases, from depression to dementia. Obesity can even rewire a baby in utero; a study published in early 2014 in the journal *Cell* showed that obesity during pregnancy may cause the fetus to develop abnormal neuronal circuits related to controlling appetite, which in turn puts the child at greater risk of weight gain and diabetes later in life.[4] Adding insult to injury, University of Oregon researchers published a paper in late 2014 showing that obesity during pregnancy harms the developing fetus's stem cells, which are responsible for creating and sustaining lifelong blood and immune-system function.[5]

For decades now scientists have been trying to come up with a solution to end obesity. Drug companies have spent billions hoping to discover a miracle pill that leads to rapid, safe weight loss without any side effects. And millions of people have emptied their wallets to purchase promising "cures"—from books and related media to supplements and dieting gimmicks—for their waistline woes. Nothing has revolutionized this industry yet. But I believe something can. And you can probably guess what that something is: tweaking the microbiome. Indeed, all the latest science points to the power of the microbiome in controlling appetite, metabolic health, and weight. Finding success in the quest to achieve optimal weight lies in whether or not you're harboring "fat" microbes.

FAT TRIBES VS. THIN TRIBES

Before I get to the details of obesity within the context of the microbiome, let's again consider the difference between the average Western child and a child from rural sub-Saharan Africa. Keep in mind that being obese or overweight is something that is virtually unheard of in this African population, compared to Western populations. Granted, some of this discrepancy is due to access to food in general, but part of the conversation now revolves around the composition of the gut bacteria in each population. In one often-cited Harvard study published in 2010, researchers looked at the effect of diet on the microbiome by evaluating the gut bacteria of children in rural Africa.[6] These children eat a high-fiber diet that is "similar to that of early human settlements at the time of the birth of agriculture." Using genetic tests, the scientists identified the types of bacteria present in the children's fecal matter. In addition, they looked at total short-chain fatty acids, which are manufactured by gut bacteria when they digest plant fiber (polysaccharides).

As we've already discussed in this book, the two largest groups of bacteria are Firmicutes and Bacteroidetes; between them, these two groups make up more than 90 percent of the gut's population. The ratio of these two groups to each other determines levels of inflammation and squarely relates to such conditions as obesity, diabetes, coronary artery disease, and inflammation in general. Although there's no perfect ratio that equates with health, we know that a higher ratio of Firmicutes to

Bacteroidetes (that is, more Firmicutes than Bacteroidetes in the gut) is strongly associated with more inflammation and more obesity.

Why? As noted earlier, Firmicutes bacteria are exceptionally adept at extracting calories from food, so they increase caloric absorption. If your body can absorb more calories from your food as it moves through the gastrointestinal tract, there's a greater likelihood of weight gain. Bacteroidetes, on the other hand, specialize in breaking down bulky plant starches and fibers into shorter fatty acid molecules that the body can use for energy. The F/B ratio is now looked upon as an "obesity biomarker."[7]

The Harvard study found that the Western guts were dominated by Firmicutes whereas the Africans' housed more Bacteroidetes. Take a look:

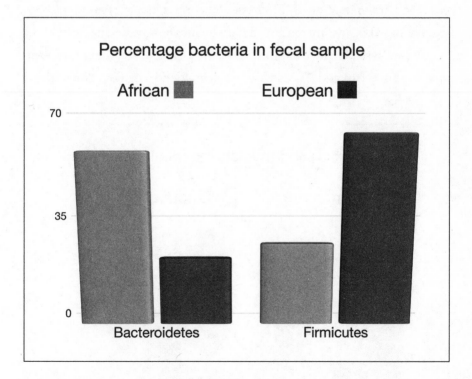

Having a gut dominated by Firmicutes has its consequences, for multiple studies have also shown that Firmicutes help regulate human metabolic genes. That means that these bacteria, which are so abundant in overweight humans, are actually controlling genes that adversely impact metabolism. They are, in essence, hijacking our DNA and creating a scenario in which our body thinks it needs to retain calories.

As the authors of a 2011 study stated, "Not only are the microorganisms increasing the energy harvest in the gut, but they are also affecting the regulation of how this energy is stored and how the immune system operates. The latter is important because imbalances in the composition of the microbial gut community can lead to inflammatory diseases, and such inflammation can be linked to obesity."[8] What's more, in early 2015 the *American Journal of Clinical Nutrition* published a study further showing that higher levels of Firmicutes changes our genetic expression, noting that this paves the way for obesity, diabetes, cardiovascular disease, and inflammation. But, as they also revealed in their study, you can change this. Just increasing dietary fiber can improve the ratio.[9]

When researchers examined the short-chain fatty acids in each group—European and African—they again found a marked difference:[10]

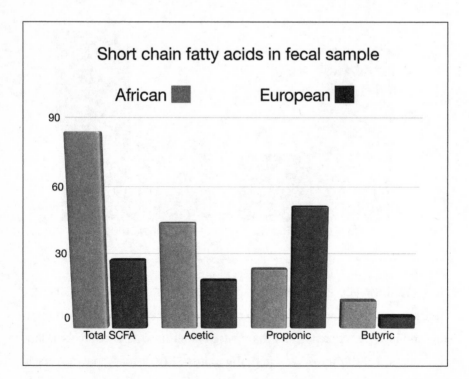

In chapter 5, we'll see what these different ratios mean. But for now we can say that you want more butyric and acetic acid and less propionic acid. High levels of propionic acid indicate that the gut is dominated by less friendly bacteria. So, indeed, the African profile reflects a much healthier microbiome than the European one. And these dissimilarities have everything to do with diet. The African diet is high in fiber and low in sugar. The European diet is the opposite. Might this help explain why obesity and even conditions like asthma aren't seen in rural Africa?

When I lecture on the topic of obesity and intestinal flora, I love sharing the recent groundbreaking 2013 study of twins published in *Science*, which was among the first of its kind to reveal the connection between the types of microbes found in the gut and the path to obesity.[11] When scientists at Washington University transferred gut bacteria from an obese human twin into the gastrointestinal tracts of slender mice, the mice grew fat. And when bacteria from the svelte twin were introduced into lean mice, the mice stayed lean so long as the animals ate a healthy diet. Earlier research had already noted remarkable differences in the array of bacteria in obese humans compared to the bacteria in those of normal weight. In one 2006 study published in *Nature*, the same Washington University group of researchers documented that obese individuals had, on average, 20 percent more Firmicutes compared to normal-weight individuals and nearly 90 percent fewer Bacteroidetes.[12] Other studies have further shown that diabetic and obese individuals tend to lack a diversity of bacteria.[13, 14] In addition, research at the Cleveland Clinic has revealed that some bacteria metabolize components of meat and eggs to produce a compound that promotes the clogging of arteries.[15] So if you have too much of this bacteria, you're at greater risk for cardiovascular disease. This might explain why some people who gorge on "artery-clogging" foods never develop heart disease whereas others with an imbalanced microbiota do. This doesn't mean you should avoid meat and eggs; on the contrary, these foods are important sources of nutrients and part of the Brain Maker program. The key point here is that imbalances in gut bacteria are root sources of health challenges. So if you're going to blame heart disease on something, the bad bugs in your belly must get part of the blame.

Before we get to the science behind the relationship between your gut's colonies and your waist size, let's review some basics that illuminate the connection between brain health and obesity—namely, the effects of high blood sugar, insulin resistance, and diabetes.

OBESITY IS AN INFLAMMATORY DISEASE, JUST LIKE BRAIN DISEASE

While it's hard to imagine obesity as an inflammatory disease, just as it may seem difficult to grasp that dementia and depression are inflammatory diseases, all are exactly that. For starters, obesity is associated with increased production of pro-inflammatory chemicals, or cytokines.[16] These molecules largely come from the fat tissue itself, which acts like an organ pumping out hormones and inflammatory substances. Fat cells do more than simply store extra calories; they are far more involved in human physiology than we had previously thought. And if you have more fat than you need, especially around visceral organs such as the liver, heart, kidneys, pancreas, and intestines, your metabolism will suffer.

This type of "visceral fat," which is often pronounced in obese individuals, spells double trouble in the body. Not only is it uniquely capable of provoking inflammatory pathways but it activates signaling molecules that can interfere with the body's normal hormonal dynamics.[17] In addition, visceral fat does more than just lead to inflammation down the road through a chain of biological events; visceral fat itself becomes inflamed. This kind of fat houses hordes of inflammatory white blood cells. What's more, when visceral fat produces hormonal and inflammatory molecules, they get dumped directly into the liver, which responds with another round of ammunition, specifically, inflammation-producing reactions and hormone-disrupting substances.

Long story short: Visceral fat is more than merely an enemy standing by. It is an enemy that is armed and dangerous. The number of health conditions now linked to visceral fat is tremendous, from the obvious ones such as obesity and metabolic syndrome to the not-so-obvious — cancer, autoimmune disorders, and brain disease. The danger of visceral fat explains why your waist size is often a measure of "health"; the roundness of your belly predicts future health challenges and mortality. Put simply, the higher your waist circumference, the higher your risk for disease and death. Girth can also predict adverse structural changes in the brain.

In another oft-cited 2005 study, a team of researchers from UC Berkeley, UC Davis, and the University of Michigan examined the waist-to-hip ratios of more than 100 individuals and compared them to structural changes in their brains as they aged.[18] They wanted to determine whether a relationship existed between the brain's structure and the size of a person's belly, and the results generated a lot of buzz in the medical community. The bigger the belly (i.e., the larger a person's waist-to-hip ratio), the smaller the brain's memory center, the hippocampus. The hippocampus's function is dependent upon its size. If your hippocampus shrinks, so does your memory.

More striking still, the researchers found that the higher the waist-to-hip ratio, the higher the risk for small strokes, which are associated with declining brain function. The authors stated: "These results are consistent with a growing body of evidence that links obesity, vascular disease, and inflammation to cognitive decline and dementia." Other studies, including one in 2010 at Boston University, have confirmed the finding: Excess pounds on the body equates with less brain volume.[19] Now, some may wish to argue the point in discussing other body parts, but when it comes to the hippocampus, size *does* matter.

Keep in mind that fat-generated cytokines are the ones found at elevated levels in all inflammatory conditions, from arthritis and heart disease to autoimmune disorders and dementia. And, as you know, we can test for inflammation through markers like C-reactive protein (CRP). As reported in the *New England Journal of Medicine*, having a high CRP level is correlated with as much as a three-fold increased risk of dementia, including Alzheimer's disease. It's also been linked to cognitive impairment and general thinking problems.[20]

So you can connect the dots: If the level of inflammation predicts neurological disorders, and excess body fat increases inflammation, obesity is a risk factor for brain disease. And such inflammation is responsible for a lot of the conditions we attribute to obesity, not just neurological challenges. It's as much a key player in diabetes as it is in hypertension, for instance. These conditions may come with separate symptoms and be categorized differently (diabetes is a metabolic problem, whereas hypertension is a cardiovascular one), but they share a key underlying feature: inflammation.

BLOOD SUGAR AND THE BRAIN

Because obesity is the outcome of metabolic dysfunction, no conversation about it can exclude the issue of blood sugar control. And I'll start this discussion with a quick look at insulin, which you already know is one of the body's most important hormones. It plays the main role in our metabolism, helping us usher energy from food into cells for their use. The process is uniquely complex. Our cells can accept glucose only with the help of insulin, which acts like a transporter and is produced by the pancreas. Insulin shuttles glucose from the bloodstream into cells, where it can then be used as fuel.

When a cell is normal and healthy, it has abundant receptors for insulin, so it has no problem responding to it. But when a cell is mercilessly exposed to high levels of insulin through a never-ending presence of glucose—caused by consuming too many carbohydrates and refined sugars—the cell does something brilliant to adapt: It reduces the number of insulin-responsive receptors on its surfaces. It's as if the cell closes a few doors so it can't hear insulin knocking. This ultimately causes the cell to become desensitized or "resistant" to insulin. Once a cell is insulin resistant, it's unable to take glucose from the blood, leaving glucose in the bloodstream. As with most biological processes, there's a "fail-safe" backup system in place. The body wants to fix this problem, as it knows it can't have glucose loitering in the blood. So it tells the pancreas to increase production of insulin to mop up that glucose, which the pancreas dutifully does. It will continue to pump out as much insulin as needed to push glucose into cells. And higher levels of insulin are needed because the cells aren't as responsive to insulin.

This, of course, sets in motion a vicious cycle that usually culminates in type 2 diabetes. By definition, a diabetic is someone who has high blood sugar because their body cannot ferry glucose into cells. And if it remains in the blood, that sugar is like an assault weapon. It inflicts a lot of damage. Diabetes is a leading cause of early death, coronary heart disease, strokes, kidney disease, blindness, and neurological disorders; we could go so far as to say it's also a major cause of Alzheimer's if it goes on untreated for years. Although most people who have type 2 diabetes are overweight, plenty of normal and even slender people are walking around today with chronic blood sugar imbalances. The road to diabetes—and, farther down that path, brain disease—starts with imbalances regardless of weight. And throughout this chain of events, the body endures a riot of inflammation.

Insulin is also a big player in the body's reactions when blood sugar levels cannot be managed well. As a so-called anabolic hormone, insulin encourages cellular growth, promotes fat formation and retention, and stimulates further inflammation. High levels of insulin rev up or turn down other hormones, thus throwing the body's overall hormonal system off balance. And this imbalance has repercussions, pushing the body further toward a biological ledge, if you will.

Surges in blood sugar have direct negative effects on the brain, effects that cause more inflammation. Blood sugar increases lead to a depletion of important neurotransmitters, including serotonin, epinephrine, norepinephrine, GABA, and dopamine. Materials needed to make these neurotransmitters, such as B-complex vitamins, also get used up. High blood sugar also causes magnesium levels to dwindle, impairing both your nervous system and liver. More important, high blood sugar sparks a reaction called "glycation," which I detailed in chapter 2. As a reminder, glycation is the biological process whereby sugar molecules bind to proteins and certain fats to form lethal new structures called AGEs, which, more than any other factor, contribute to the degeneration of the brain and its functioning. This process can even lead to the shrinking of critical brain tissue. In fact, scientists now understand that insulin resistance can precipitate the formation of those infamous plaques that are present in Alzheimer's brains. Remember that those with diabetes are at least twice as likely to develop Alzheimer's disease and that obese people are at a much greater risk of impaired brain function.

To be sure, diabetes doesn't directly cause Alzheimer's disease. But the two share the same origin: diabetes and Alzheimer's both result from a dietary onslaught to the body that forces it to adapt by developing biological pathways that eventually lead to dysfunction and, later on, illness. Diabetes and even slight blood sugar issues below the threshold for diabetes are directly associated with increased risk for brain shrinkage and Alzheimer's disease. The parallel rise in the number of people with type 2 diabetes, obesity, and Alzheimer's in the past decade is undoubtedly connected.

But what's causing all the diabetes? The data showing the relationship between high carbohydrate consumption and diabetes is almost indisputable. In 1994, when the American Diabetes Association recommended that Americans consume 60 to 70 percent of their calories from carbohydrates, the diabetes (and obesity) epidemic took off. Between 1997 and 2007 the number of cases of diabetes in the U.S. doubled. From 1980 through 2011, the number more than *tripled*. As of 2014, the Centers for Disease Control and Prevention estimates that more than 29 million Americans—one out of every eleven people—has diabetes, and nearly 28 percent of those people don't even know they have it—they are undiagnosed.[21] I think it's safe to say the number of prediabetics—those who are starting to have blood sugar imbalances but don't know it—has similarly skyrocketed.

BLAME THE BUGS, NOT THE BONBONS

Make no mistake: blood sugar regulation is priority #1 when it comes to preserving brain function and resisting Alzheimer's disease. And blood sugar levels reflect not just dietary sugar and carbohydrate consumption, but also the balance of bacteria in the gut. New research performed in just the past few years is telling us that certain types of gut bacteria actually help the body control blood sugar levels. (I'll get to the details of the latest studies shortly.)

Research is underway examining how certain probiotics might be able to reverse type 2 diabetes and the neurological challenges that can follow. At Harvard's 2014 symposium on the microbiome, I was floored by the work of Dr. M. Nieuwdorp from the University of Amsterdam, who has done some incredible research related to obesity and type 2 diabetes.[22] He has successfully improved the blood sugar mayhem found in type 2 diabetes in more than 250 people using fecal transplantation. He's also used this procedure to improve insulin sensitivity.

These two achievements are virtually unheard of in traditional medicine. We have no medication available to reverse diabetes or significantly improve insulin sensitivity. Dr. Nieuwdorp had the room riveted, practically silenced, by his presentation. In this experiment, he transplanted fecal material from a healthy, lean, nondiabetic into a dia-betic. What he did to control his experiment was quite clever: He simply transplanted the participants' own microbiome back into their colons, so they didn't know whether they were being "treated" or not. For those of us who see the far-reaching effects of diabetes in patients on a daily basis, outcomes like Dr. Nieuwdorp's are a beacon of hope. And as a neurologist who recognizes the profound relationship between elevated blood sugar and brain degeneration, I believe this groundbreaking research opens the door to a whole new world of possibilities in terms of preventing and even treating brain disorders.

Each day it seems a new diet or supplement appears that promises to help with weight loss. Obese people are blamed for their own weight issues, because it seems they cannot restrain themselves from eating the foods that we know are associated with weight gain. Generally, we acknowledge that the modern Western diet, high in carbohydrates and refined sugars as well as processed fat, is responsible for the obesity epi-demic. We also tend to think that people who are overweight are lazy and don't burn enough calories relative to what they take in.

But what if being overweight or obese has less to do with willpower or even genetic forces and more to do with the microbial profile in the gut? What if we owe our obesity challenges to a sick and dysfunctional congregation of intestinal bugs?

Millions of people will be relieved to know that their weight gain may not be their fault. New research shows that our gut bacteria don't just aid in digestion, as you likely realize by now. They play a critical role in our metabolism, and this relates directly to whether we lose or gain weight. Because they influence the way we store fat, balance levels of glucose in the blood, express genes that relate to metabolism, and respond to hormones that make us feel hungry or full, gut bacteria are the masters of ceremonies in a lot of ways. From the moment of our birth, they help set the stage for whether we become obese, diabetic, and brain sick or lean and mean with a healthy, quick-thinking brain and a long, robust lifespan.

It's now firmly established that the gut community of lean people resembles a rainforest filled with many species and that of obese people is much less diverse. We used to think that being overweight or obese was a math problem—a factor of excess caloric intake compared to calories expended. But this new research reveals that the microbiome plays a fundamental role in our body's energy dynamics, which affects the calories-in/calories-out equation. If you house too many types of bacteria that can efficiently remove more calories from your food, guess what: you'll absorb more calories than you probably need, leading to fat promotion.

To get a better sense of how scientists managed to document microbial differences between lean and fat people and correlate that with obesity, it helps to take a closer look at the research of Jeffrey Gordon of Washington University in St. Louis.[23] He and his colleagues are among the scientists conducting groundbreaking experiments with "humanized" mice. In his now-famous 2013 twins study I previously mentioned, Gordon once again showed the power of "fat" versus "thin" tribes dominating in the gut and risk for obesity.[24] After his team engineered baby mice to contain microbes from either an obese woman or her lean twin, they let the mice eat the same diet in equal amounts. And that's when they observed that the mice soon parted ways in terms of their heaviness. The animals that acquired bacteria from an obese woman not only grew fatter than the mice with microbes from a thin woman, but their gut microbes were much less diverse.

The experiment was then repeated, but this time Gordon's team let the baby mice share the same cage after they'd been engineered to have either "fat" or "lean" microbes in their guts. This allowed the mice carrying microbes from the obese woman to acquire some of the microbes from their lean roommates, mostly through consuming the feces of the lean mice—a typical mouse behavior. The result? Both sets of mice remained lean. Gordon took his experiment further by transferring strains of bacteria from the lean mice to those destined to become obese, which instead developed a healthy weight. Gordon was quoted as saying, "Taken together, these experiments provide pretty compelling proof that there is a cause-and-effect relationship and that it was possible to prevent the development of obesity."[25]

How do Gordon and his team make sense of this? He posits that the gut bacteria in obese mice are missing microbes that have starring roles in maintaining a normal metabolism and healthy body weight. His studies, alongside those of others, are providing new information about what those roles entail. For example, one such missing microbe that's associated with regulating hunger is *Helicobacter pylori*, which helps control appetite by affecting levels of ghrelin, the main hormone that stimulates appetite. *H. pylori* enjoyed a symbiotic relationship with us in our guts for at least the past 58,000 years, but our Western digestive tracts no longer include very much of it because of our hygienic living conditions and profligate use of antibiotics.

Gordon's team is among the pioneering scientists who are also making the connections among quality of the diet, quality and diversity of the gut bacteria, and risk for becoming obese. Using mouse models again, he has shown that when you feed humanized mice a "Western diet" — one that's low in fiber, fruits, and vegetables but high in fat, the mice with obese-type microbes become obese even when exposed to their lean counterparts. In other words, the unhealthy diet prevents the "slenderizing" bacteria from moving in and having a positive impact. Such results further point to the power of diet in controlling the composition of the gut bacteria and, ultimately, weight control. Clearly, more studies are needed, especially using humans, but Gordon's research has nonetheless attracted a lot of attention in health circles and inspired further investigations.

In 2013, another team of researchers, this one from MIT and the Aristotle University of Thessaloniki in Greece, added to the evidence when they examined why a probiotic-filled yogurt could have such a powerful slimming effect.[26] They fed mice a range of diets, but these weren't your average mice; they were genetically predisposed to obesity. The mice that ate a "fast food" diet—one high in unhealthy fat and sugar and low in fiber and vitamins B and D—quickly grew obese. Their gut microbes changed after just a few weeks of dining on the fast food. In contrast, the mice that got three servings per week of commercially available probiotic yogurt remained lean. But here's the kicker: these yogurt-eating mice were also allowed to eat as much fast food as they wanted! The headline of their results said it all: "Eating Westernized 'Fast Food' Style Diet Restructures the Gut Microbiome and Accelerates Age-Associated Obesity in Mice," and "Dietary Supplementation with Probiotic Yogurt Inhibits Obesity." Obviously, I don't want to give the impression that taking probiotics gives you free license to eat whatever you choose, but the research does have huge implications.

One of the most insidious villains with respect to our gut's microbiome, which I've briefly mentioned and will explore in further detail later, is processed fructose. The typical American consumes high-fructose corn syrup at the rate of 132 to 312 calories a day.[27] (I'll further point out that consumption of this product has steadily increased in parallel with the growing rate of obesity.) Many scientists have suggested that processed fructose is contributing to the obesity epidemic and that it is one of the biggest factors in creating a so-called Westernized gut microbiome, that is, one with little diversity and too many types of bacteria that feed fat cells.

Why is fructose particularly offensive? Not only does it feed pathogenic gut bacteria, thereby disrupting a healthy microbial balance, but fructose does not stimulate insulin production as glucose does. It's immediately handled by the liver, and this means the body's production of leptin, another important hormone related to appetite suppression, goes down. You don't feel full, so you keep eating. This same outcome—a lack of satiety—is also seen with artificial sweeteners. Although we used to think that sugar substitutes like saccharin, sucralose, and aspartame didn't have a metabolic impact because they don't raise insulin, it turns out that they can indeed wreak tremendous metabolic havoc and cause the same metabolic disorders as real sugar. How so? They do this by changing the microbiome in ways that favor dysbiosis, blood sugar imbalances, and an overall unhealthy metabolism. And yes, the food and beverage industry has a splitting headache over this latest study, which was published in 2014 in the journal *Nature*.[28] I'll get to the details of this study in chapter 6, for it provides the evidence that the gut bacteria are responsible for helping to control blood sugar control and, in turn, weight and risk for disease.

WHY GASTRIC BYPASS WORKS: THANK YOUR BUGS

Drastic approaches to weight loss, such as gastric bypass surgery, which physically reorganizes the digestive system, have become increasingly popular. These surgeries often involve making the stomach smaller and rerouting the small intestine. And while we used to think that they triggered rapid weight loss largely by forcing the person to consume less, a monumental study published in *Nature* in 2014 put forth the idea that the microbiome determines the success of gastric surgery.[29] We now have astonishing new evidence that a major portion of the weight loss is credited to changes in the gut microbiota. These changes happen after surgery in response to not just the anatomical changes but the dietary shifts that typically occur as the person consumes healthier foods that favor the growth of different bacteria. I have no doubt that when we ferret out the details as to why diabetic gastric bypass patients also often experience a complete reversal of their diabetes soon after surgery, we will yet again find ourselves looking at the microbiome.

As we've discussed, the ratio of bacteria types in the gut is important. Multiple studies show that when the number of Firmicutes is reduced, so is the risk for metabolic problems like diabetes. On the other hand, when the number of Bacteroidetes is low, there is increased gut permeability, which in turn raises all kinds of risks, not the least of which is immune system mayhem, inflammation, and, farther down the road, brain-related disorders and diseases, from depression to Alzheimer's.

I should also add that exercise serves a role in promoting the right balance of microbes. We've long known about the benefits of exercise in general, but it turns out that its impact in weight loss and management isn't just about burning more calories. New science reveals that exercise positively influences the gut's balance of bacteria to favor colonies that prevent weight gain. In laboratory studies of mice, higher levels of exercise correlated with a reduction in Firmicutes and an increase in Bacteroidetes. In other words, exercise effectively lowered the F/B ratio. Although more human studies are needed and are currently under way, we already have compelling evidence that the same holds true in us. Exercise fosters a diverse microbiome.

In 2014, researchers at Ireland's University College Cork examined blood and stool samples to compare the difference between the microbial diversity in professional rugby players and healthy, nonathlete men.[30] Some of the nonathletes were of normal weight and some were overweight. (The blood tests provided information about muscle damage and inflammation — signs of how much exercise the men had done recently.) Overall, the forty athletes they studied showed greater diversity of microbes than any of the other men who participated in the experiment. In their paper, published in *Gut*, the researchers attributed these results to the athletes' strenuous exercise and to their diets, which were higher in protein (22 percent of calories from protein versus 15 to 16 percent consumed by the nonathletes). Another key finding here was that in addition to documenting a richer diversity of gut microbes in the athletes, the researchers reported that among the microbes seen in these rugby players was a strain of bacteria linked with lower rates of obesity and obesity-related disorders.

The science is speaking for itself: From the day we are born, the interaction between gut bacteria and our diet can make us vulnerable to metabolic dysfunction and brain disease. It's no longer a mystery to me and my colleagues in medicine why babies who are not exposed to a rich array of beneficial bacteria in early life go on to live with a much higher risk for obesity, diabetes, and neurological challenges than their peers who develop healthier microbiomes. These at-risk babies are typically the ones delivered by elective C-section, are mostly formula-fed, and often suffer from chronic infections for which antibiotics are prescribed. In one particularly illuminating study, Canadian researchers discovered that formula-fed babies develop certain strains of bacteria in their gut that breast-fed babies don't develop until they start eating solid foods.[31] These strains are not necessarily pathogenic, but early exposure to certain types of bacteria might not be a good thing since an infant's gut and immune system are still maturing, a fact echoed by researchers in this area who agree that this could be one reason formula-fed babies are more suscepti-ble to autoimmune conditions such as asthma, allergies, eczema, and celiac disease, as well as obesity.

That said, let me briefly address the women who do use formula. For some, breastfeeding just isn't an option. Or a woman may choose or need to wean early. Does this mean she is dooming her child? Not in the least. While we know that breast-fed babies have a much more diverse microbi-ome and reduced risk for a medley of health conditions than babies who are formula-fed, we also know that there's a lot you can do to support the development of a healthy microbiome in the absence of breastfeeding. You'll rejoice at just how receptive the microbiome is to rehabilitation through basic lifestyle shifts. I'll be giving moms some ideas about how to do this in chapter 8.

Concerns about the extravagant use of antibiotics in children have only intensified in light of the childhood obesity epidemic. We now have plenty of evidence to blame the obesity epidemic partly on the use of antibiotics and their role in changing the balance of gut microbes. Dr. Martin Blaser of N.Y.U.'s Microbiome Project has also demonstrated that when young mice receive low doses of antibiotics, similar to the amount livestock receive, they pack on 15 percent more body fat than mice that aren't exposed to such drugs.[32] Think about that, and consider the following: The average American child receives three courses of antibiotics during the first year of life. Blaser made this point very clear during his presentation at Harvard's Probiotics Symposium in 2014.

In the cogent words of researcher Dr. Maria Gloria Dominguez-Bello, also of N.Y.U. (and married to Dr. Blaser), "Antibiotics are like a fire in the forest. The baby is forming a forest. If you have a fire in a forest that is new, you get extinction."[33]

In a related study, when a graduate student in Blaser's laboratory fed mice both a high-fat diet and antibiotics, the mice became obese, results that point to a "synergy" going on between the antibiotics and the diet.[34] Interestingly, Blaser notes that antibiotic use varies greatly across the U.S. and that when you look at a map, you can see a pattern: In the states where obesity rates are highest, so is antibiotic use. And the South wins the award for being the most overweight and overprescribed.

Before you feel overwhelmed by this information and close the book, especially as it may pertain to your own life, let me be clear: What all this astonishing new data means is that you can control your metabolism and, in turn, your inflammatory pathways and brain health just by nourishing your microbiome. Even if you weren't blessed by being born by a vaginal delivery and even if you've taken antibiotics before (and who hasn't?) or eaten a carb-rich diet, I have solutions that will help you to turn the train around.

I'll get to all of the practical strategies soon. For now, let's turn to one more condition that's on everyone's mind: autism spectrum disorder. At last, in the 21st century we may find some preventive measures against and better, individualized treatments for this neurological challenge in some individuals. Although many questions remain about this enigmatic brain disorder, the role of the intestinal microbiome is becoming increasingly obvious. The latest science is, as you're about to find out, laying the foundation for a new frontier in medicine.

CHAPTER 5

Autism and the Gut

On the Frontiers of Brain Medicine

HARDLY A DAY GOES BY that I don't answer a question about autism, one of the most debated disorders in the last decade. What exactly causes it? Why are so many children diagnosed with it today? Will there ever be a cure or guaranteed preventive measure? Why is there such a broad range in severity? Nearly sixty years after the disorder was first identified, the number of cases continues to rise. The United Nations estimates that up to 70 million people worldwide fall on the autism spectrum, three million of whom are in the U.S.[1]

First, let me clarify that for purposes of this discussion, I'm going to use to term *autism* to encompass all the degrees on the spectrum. To be sure, *autism spectrum disorder* (ASD) and *autism* are both general terms to describe a large and diverse family of complex disorders of brain development. These disorders share three classic characteristics: difficulties in social interaction, challenges with verbal and nonverbal communication, and repetitive behaviors. According to the Centers for Disease Control and Prevention (CDC), children or adults with autism might[2]

- not point at objects to show interest (for example, not point at an airplane flying overhead)

- not look at objects when another person points at them

- have trouble relating to others or lack interest in other people

- avoid eye contact and prefer to be alone

- have trouble understanding other people's feelings or talking about their own feelings

- prefer not to be held or cuddled, or might cuddle only when *they* want to

- be unresponsive when people talk to them, but respond to other sounds

- be very interested in people, but not know how to talk, play with, or relate to them

- repeat or echo words or phrases said to them, or repeat words or phrases in place of normal language

- have trouble using typical words or motions to express their needs

- not play typical "pretend" games (for example, pretending to feed a doll)

- repeat actions over and over again

- have trouble adapting when a routine changes

- have unusual reactions to the way things smell, taste, look, feel, or sound

- lose skills they once had (for example, might stop saying words they previously used)

Although distinct subtypes were once recognized, including Asperger's syndrome and autistic disorder, in 2013 all autism disorders were merged under one big umbrella diagnosis of ASD. But no two individuals are absolutely alike; one person can have a mild case and be socially awkward but excel in math or art, for example, while another can struggle with motor coordination, have intellectual deficits, and experience severe physical health issues such as insomnia and chronic diarrhea and constipation. Dr. Stephen Scherer, who directs the Centre for Applied Genomics at Toronto's Hospital for Sick Children and the McLaughlin Centre at the University of Toronto, and who just completed the largest-ever autism genome study, uses an apt analogy: "Each child with autism is like a snowflake—unique from the others."[3] His latest study has revealed that the disorder's genetic underpinnings are even more complex than previously thought. Contrary to what scientists long assumed, most siblings who share the same biological parents and a diagnosis of autism don't always have the same autism-linked genes.[4] This study has raised new suspicions about the disorder, including the possibility that autism isn't usually inherited, even when it runs in families.

Despite the dramatic differences among people with autism, one thing is for sure: They reflect a community of people whose brains function a little differently. During their early brain development, something triggered changes in their physiology and neurology that led to the disorder. Now that autism is so prevalent, with such wide parameters, there has been a cultural shift in how we think about it. Some choose to refer to the condition, especially in regard to high-functioning individuals with autism, as more of a personality style as opposed to an illness. This is similar to how many members of the deaf community do not consider themselves disabled, but simply people with different modes of communication. I appreciate this shift to a humanistic perspective, though I don't know any parent of a child with autism who would choose to avoid a cure or effective treatment if there was one. Even those children with exceptional abilities in visual skills, music, and academics can have their challenges.

Whether we view autism as a personality style or as an illness, there's no denying that it's sharply on the rise. Signs and symptoms of autism tend to emerge when children are between two and three years of age, though some doctors can spot signs in that first year of life. One in 68 American children is on the autism spectrum. This reflects a tenfold increase in prevalence over the past forty years—a surge too great to be justified solely by the fact that people are more aware of autism and seeking diagnoses. One in 42 boys and one in 189 girls is affected, making autism four to five times more common in boys than in girls. In America, more than 2 million individuals are officially diagnosed. I know I'm not the only one calling this an epidemic. Take a look at the following chart showing the rise in cases from 1970 to 2013:[5]

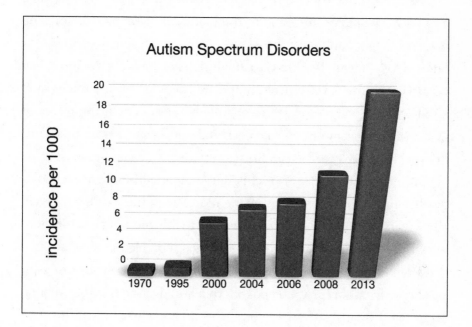

A few years ago, I would not have touched the subject of autism. It was just too fraught; the conversation was mired in the controversy about the vaccine-autism connection, a connection that has been scientifically disproven.[6] At that time, we were still in the blind era of saying "I don't know" to the question of what causes autism. Some found it easier to place full blame on vaccines than to examine other, seemingly improbable contributors to the condition, such as an unhealthy microbiome. But today, a lot has changed. Legitimate studies from top institutions are currently uncovering the gut-bug connection to the disorder. Research is now delivering surprising and encouraging answers. What scientists are finding out today about autism has implications that go far beyond understanding and addressing that condition. Contrary to popular wisdom, the latest science in this realm overlaps significantly with that concerning other neurological ailments. Researching autism means being on the frontiers of brain medicine, especially as the science relates to an understanding of the microbiome.

As I've described, for a long time problems with the gut were regarded as a set of symptoms unrelated to the brain, but we're now discovering how gut health and function—especially gut bacteria—connect to brain development. We are also finally seeing how gut bacteria may contribute to the development and progression of a brain disorder such as autism.[7] As you'll soon learn, one of the most convincing pieces of evidence linking intestinal microbes and autism is the fact that children with autism exhibit certain patterns in the composition of their gut bacteria that are absent in children without autism.[8] For a neurologist like me, who helps parents treat children with this baffling disorder, this observation is a huge red flag, coupled with the fact that individuals with autism almost uniformly suffer from GI problems.

Moreover, the particular species of gut bacteria often seen in individuals with autism create compounds that are adversarial to the immune system and brain—they can rouse the immune system and increase inflammation. In a young person whose brain is rapidly developing, exposure to these compounds in addition to the increased inflammation may very well play a role in a brain disorder like autism. The scientists on the frontiers of this research, some of whom you'll meet in this chapter, are currently studying the relationships between the gut bacteria, their byproducts, and the risk of autism. This research is also looking at the roles of the immune and nervous systems—two key players in the development of any neurological disorder.

Just as there is no single type of autism, there is no single cause. Scientists, for example, have identified a multitude of rare gene changes, or mutations, associated with autism. In fact, as I write this, two sweeping new studies have shown links between more than 100 genes and the disorder.[9, 10] These mutations appear to disrupt the brain's nerve network, and they don't all come from Mom and Dad—many of these mutations can occur spontaneously in the egg or sperm right before conception.

While a small number of these mutations are probably sufficient to cause autism by themselves, most cases of autism—as with most conditions and disorders—are likely caused by a combination of autism risk genes and environmental factors influencing early brain development. Which also helps explain why biological siblings with autism don't necessarily carry the same autism risk genes. Something else is also going on from an environmental standpoint. From what I've witnessed in my practice and culled from the latest research, my guess is that the environmental impact is greater than the genetic one. Just as changes in the gut bacteria can affect an individual's healthy immunology and neurology, contributing to the risk of conditions like MS and dementia, so too can such changes translate to a higher probability of autism in a developing child. After all, most kids with autism have an early life history of at least one or two traumas, hence the headlines you read in health magazines, such as "Preeclampsia During Mother's Pregnancy Associated with Greater Autism Risk," "Use of Drug X During Pregnancy Associated with Increased Risk of Autism," "Kids Born Pre-Term at Increased Risk of Developing Autism," "Maternal Inflammation Linked to Autism in Offspring," and so on. These events not only influence a child's developing immune system and brain, but, should the child miss out on that microbial baptism at birth and go on to face multiple infections for which antibiotics are used, the developing microbiome will be greatly affected. And because these impacts begin in utero, figuring out exactly when any given individual's "switch" for autism gets turned on is difficult—if not impossible—to know. By the time a child is diagnosed with autism, he or she has been exposed to a lot of potential disorder triggers in his or her unique body, and the development of autism clearly reflects a confluence of forces. Future research will bear this out, but I wouldn't be surprised to find that many people carry the genetic risk factors for autism *but never develop it* because the genes are never given the opportunity to express themselves. In other words, the genes may be silenced by their environment. This is true for many health conditions, in fact. You could carry genes that put you at a much higher risk for obesity, heart disease, and dementia than someone who doesn't have underlying genetic susceptibilities, yet you may never suffer from these maladies because the genes remain dormant due to their environment.

In this chapter, we're going to take a tour of this mysterious condition, autism. I will present the latest facts and the correlations that science has made, some of which continue to emerge as I write this. The science relating autism to changes in the gut bacteria is clearly in its early stages and is evolving quickly. I am compelled to share what we know because the reports thus far are so powerful and hopeful, and I believe that the many people who are desperate for answers and guidance deserve to hear them. I am confident that the clues surfacing today will eventually be proven in the kinds of rigorous, large-scale human studies that lead to meaningful treatments for many people with the disorder. All I ask is that you be open to a new perspective that you might not have heard before. My guess is that you'll leave this chapter feeling empowered in ways you didn't expect, even if you never have to face a diagnosis of autism in a loved one. Much of this information reinforces an important takeaway of this book: the power—and vulnerability—of the microbiome. (For ongoing updates on this subject, please go to my website at www.DrPerlmutter.com.)

THE STORY OF JASON

Before I get to the specifics of the gut-autism connection, let me detail a case that's emblematic of what I've witnessed in some of my own patients with the brain disorder. Although this one may sound extreme, it reflects what I've routinely begun to experience in my practice, and I know that I'm not alone. I've spoken with colleagues who are now recommending treatment protocols similar to the one you're about to hear about, which have resulted in stunning outcomes. As you read about Jason, make mental notes of the events in his life that could have impacted his microbiome. This will prime you to grasp the finer details of the connection between a dysfunctional gut and dysfunctional brain.

Twelve-year-old Jason was brought to see me by his mother because he was deemed to be on the autistic spectrum. My first order of business was to get a full history of his life up to that point. I learned that Jason had been born naturally but that his mother had taken a daily dose of antibiotics during her entire third trimester for "persistent bladder infections." Shortly after Jason's birth, he also began taking multiple courses of antibiotics for persistent ear infections. His mother said that during his first year of life he was on antibiotics "more often than not." She also shared that Jason had been a colicky baby, crying all the time in his first month. Because of his chronic ear infections, tubes were eventually placed in his ears. This procedure had to be done twice. When Jason was two, a period of chronic diarrhea led to a suspicion of celiac disease, but this was never confirmed. By the time Jason was four, he'd taken multiple rounds of antibiotics for various infections, including strep throat. Some of his illnesses were so severe that doctors delivered the antibiotics by injection.

Jason's parents became concerned about developmental issues when he was thirteen to fourteen months old. They began occupational as well as physical therapy. Jason had an extreme delay in his ability to speak; at three years old he could use sign language but speak only single words.

As you would expect, his parents had taken him to multiple doctors through the years and collected quite a library of data. There'd been EEG monitoring, MRI scans of his brain, and an assortment of blood studies, all of which were unrevealing. Jason developed obsessions with things like turning lights on and off, as well as repetitive hand movements. He lacked social skills and would not interact with others to any significant degree. His mother also said that when Jason was placed in an environment where he felt unsteady or that would challenge his balance, he'd become anxious and uncomfortable.

I noticed during my review of Jason's medical records that there were multiple entries by his treating physicians over the years not just for throat and ear infections requiring antibiotics, but also for gastrointestinal issues. "Stomach ache," for example, appeared as a common reason for office visits. On one occasion he was in the doctor's office for "projectile vomiting."

When I examined Jason, he passed his neurological examination easily. He showed good coordination, solid balance, and a normal ability to walk and run. During the course of his exam, though, he did appear anxious and would wring his hands in a repetitive manner. He could not remain seated for any meaningful length of time, he couldn't keep focused eye contact with me as I examined him, and he couldn't speak to me in full sentences.

When I sat down with his mother and discussed my findings and recommendations, I first confirmed the autism diagnosis but then quickly dived into how we could begin to address Jason's challenges. I spent a lot of time describing the impact of his exposure to antibiotics, both before birth and thereafter. I described the role of gut bacteria in controlling inflammation and regulating brain function, as well as how recent research had clearly revealed a correlation between autism and the type of bacteria found in the gut. Although I was careful not to pin Jason's autism on any single causative trigger, impressing upon his mother that the condition is likely the result of a constellation of both genetic and environmental factors, I emphasized the importance of doing all that we could to control as many variables as possible that could potentially have an impact on his brain's functionality. And that, of course, included the state of Jason's microbiome. Knowing that the current research—

some of which I'll describe shortly—was showing patterns in the gut bacteria of individuals with autism and that the microbiome could have a big influence on neurobehavioral development, I had my starting point for offering solutions. It would focus on Jason's gut.

I didn't feel it was necessary to perform a lot of laboratory studies on Jason, but I did order a stool analysis to get a sense of his gut's health. And that's when I discovered what I thought would be true: Jason's gut had virtually no *Lactobacillus* species, an indication of serious trauma to the microbiome.

My first follow-up with Jason's mother was three weeks later. At this point he had begun aggressive oral probiotics and vitamin D. She had good news to report: Jason's anxiety had diminished considerably, and he was able to tie his own shoes for the first time. Incredibly, he was able to ride a roller coaster and, also for the first time, able to spend the night away from home. Five weeks later his mother reported that his improvements had persisted but she was curious to try fecal transplantation to reap more gains in his health. She was already quite educated on this subject and had clearly done her homework.

Fecal microbial transplant (FMT) is the most aggressive therapy available to reset and recolonize a very sick microbiome. As you'll recall, it's the therapy Carlos used to treat his multiple sclerosis. (I'll explain it in greater detail in the epilogue, where I cover the future of medicine; as mentioned, FMT is not widely available in the U.S., and it's reserved for treating certain *Clostridium difficile* [C. *diff*] infections only. But this is likely to change, given the accumulating data on its utility and effectiveness in treating an array of disorders, especially those of the neurological system.)

Before you jump to conclusions about this procedure, whose unpleasant-sounding name leaves much to the imagination, let me explain what FMT entails. Much in the way we treat liver or kidney failure with transplantation, we now have an incredibly effective way of reestablishing the balance and diversity of the gut's microbiome: by transplanting good bacteria from a healthy person into the colon of another person. We do so by extracting fecal material in which the good bacteria thrive and introducing it into the diseased gut. (For the record, I do not perform fecal transplants, but I do provide information about clinics that conduct them; this is a rapidly growing industry that requires careful research on the part of the patient and donor before proceeding, as well as experienced practitioners. See the epilogue for more details.) Jason's mother went ahead with the fecal transplant, using a friend's healthy daughter as a donor.

My next contact with the family came in the form of a video that was sent to my cell phone while I was lecturing in Germany about a month later. This brief video clip took my breath away and brought tears to my eyes. It showed a vibrant, happy Jason jumping up and down on a trampoline, speaking much more engagingly with his mother than ever before. There was no text accompanying the video, nor did there need to be.

When I returned from Germany, I again caught up with Jason's mother over the phone. Here is a snapshot of what she described to me: "Jason is so much more talkative and conversational and in fact he now initiates conversation himself. There is no more handwringing and he doesn't talk to himself anymore. He is so calm and interactive. The other day he sat in a chair for 40 minutes talking to me while I was getting my hair done. I've never seen him do this.... And we've gotten the report from his teacher saying that Jason is now 'present' and very conversational. For the first time ever he's singing hymns in church, and we feel very blessed.... Thank you for helping to heal my son."

Don't get me wrong: I am not suggesting that fecal transplantation is a sure-fire remedy for all who have been diagnosed with autism, but results like this inspire me to continue trying this therapy on patients with autism in the hopes that some may benefit. After all, there is solid science supporting the role of alterations in the gut microbiome as an important factor in this disorder. And in my own clinical experience, rebuilding the gut microbiome from the ground up is working.

Jason's response to the combination of my protocol and the FMT was healing for both himself and his family. The video that Jason's mother sent me illustrated the paradigm shift in our ability to treat autism. My conversations with her now center upon what more can be done so that others can learn about this new perspective on treating autism. As such, she has given me permission to write about Jason's case not only in this book but also on my website, and has even allowed me to share the video demonstrating his incredible recovery, which I've posted on my website at www.DrPerlmutter.com/BrainMaker.

GUT DYSFUNCTION CONTRIBUTING TO BRAIN DYSFUNCTION

Multiple studies now show that GI conditions are among the hallmarks of autism. Parents of children with autism usually report that their children suffer from abdominal pain, constipation, diarrhea, and bloating. In 2012, researchers at the National Institutes of Health evaluated children with autism and found that constipation was seen in 85 percent of them, with gastrointestinal distress noted in 92 percent.[11] The main purpose of the study was to answer this question: Do children with autism actually have GI issues, or is that a mistaken observation on the part of the parents? The concluding notes by these researchers stated, "This study validates parental concerns for gastrointestinal dysfunction in children with autistic spectrum disorder." They further indicated that they had found a "strong association between constipation and language impairment." Today, the CDC estimates that children with autism are more than 3.5 times more likely to experience chronic diarrhea and constipation than their peers who do not have autism—a statistic that just cannot be ignored.

Other research has determined that another pattern exists among many individuals with autism: leaky gut.[12] As you know, this can result in an overly active immune response and inflammation that reaches the brain. One 2010 study even found a pattern of higher levels of LPS—the pro-inflammatory molecule—in patients with severe autism.[13] LPS, you'll recall, should generally not find its way to the bloodstream but can do so if the intestinal wall is compromised. Due to findings like these, many experts, including me, now recommend a diet that won't threaten that intestinal wall (i.e., gluten-free) for children with autism.

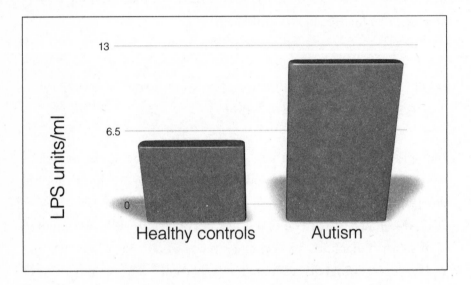

Studies have also shown increased lymphoid tissue in as many as 93 percent of patients with autism.[14] Part of the immune system, much of this tissue is found in the loose connective-tissue spaces beneath epithelial membranes, such as those that line the gastrointestinal tract and the respiratory system. Scientists can view this abnormality, which can extend from a patient's esophagus down through the large intestine.

Clearly, a lot is going on in the guts of people with autism. If we take a step back and ask what might be causing all these issues, we have to consider the microbiome. Cutting-edge research is finding that the gut ecosystem of individuals with autism is dramatically different from that of people without autism.[15] In particular, people with autism tend to have higher levels of clostridial species, which crowd out the balancing effects of other gut bacteria, leading to lower levels of beneficial bugs like bifido-bacteria.[16, 17] Higher levels of clostridial species may help explain why many kids with autism crave carbohydrates—especially refined sugars, the foods that feed these bugs—creating a vicious cycle that fuels the proliferation of more Clostridia.

The most famous clostridial species of bacteria is C. *diff*, which I briefly covered in chapter 1. When it's allowed to overgrow, it can be deadly. Certain antibiotics, chiefly fluoroquinolones and sulfur-based antibiotics as well as certain cephalosporins, can trigger such an over-growth and throw the overall balance of intestinal bacteria off-kilter. Ironically, treating a C. *diff* infection often entails the use of vancomy-cin, another antibiotic that again changes the balance of gut bacteria, killing the C. *diff*, and is not absorbed by the gut. In fact, high-profile studies have shown that in some children with autism, treatment with oral vancomycin can result in impressive improvements in behavioral, cognitive, and gastrointestinal symptoms of the disorder in some patients.[18, 19] Which raises the question: Are some species of Clostridia a potential causative agent in many cases of autism? Or, if these bugs don't cause autism, could they be increasing the risk of autism, contributing to its development, driving some of the symptoms, and exacerbating the condition once it's established? One more possibility that science needs to investigate is whether the disruptions in the gut bacteria are a result, rather than a causative agent, of the autism. Whatever the answers to these important questions are, a simple truth remains: The research thus far showing the power of leveraging the microbiome to lessen symptoms of autism is spectacular in many instances of the disorder.

The correlation between the overgrowth of potentially pathogenic bacteria and autism was first proposed in 2000 in a paper published in the *Journal of Child Neurology* by Dr. Richard Sandler and his colleagues.[20] Dr. Sandler had led a pilot study of antibiotic treatment in eleven chil-dren diagnosed with autism. Although a small number of children were involved in the study, which was carried out at the Rush-Presbyterian-St. Luke's Medical Center in Chicago, it nonetheless took the medical world by storm. It was the first study of its kind to present evidence that disruption in gut bacteria may cause certain cases of autism and that treating the disruption can significantly alleviate the symptoms of autism. In the paper, Dr. Sandler and his team describe the case of Andy Bolte, whose mother, Ellen, suspected that her son's autism was linked to a bacterial infection in his gut. She'd apparently been doing her own review of the medical literature. Andy was diagnosed with autism in 1994, following normal development until he was treated with antibiotics for an ear infection at age 18 months. Ellen had a hunch the antibiotics wiped out his gut's good bacteria, allowing the bad bacteria to thrive. In 1996, Ellen Bolte finally tested her hypothesis with the help of a doctor willing to treat her son with the same antibiotic used to treat C. *diff*, thereby bringing the balance back to his gut bacteria. Andy improved immediately and his story became the highlight of a documentary called *The Autism Enigma*, which aired overseas and was made available in the U.S. in 2012.

Other studies have since found similar findings. Dr. Sydney Finegold, an emeritus professor of medicine at UCLA who was among the co-authors of Dr. Sandler's pioneering study, ran another small trial with ten children diagnosed with autism. His group found that eight of them showed improved behavior and communication skills with the same drug treatment, and then relapsed after the treatment ended.[21] Dr. Finegold has repeatedly found that the number of clostridial species in the stools of children with autism is much greater than in the stools of children without autism (who are the controls used in the studies).[22] In one such study, children with autism had nine species of *Clostridium* not found in the controls, whereas the controls yielded only three species not identified in children with autism.

To understand the connection between high levels of clostridial species and autism, we need to understand the role that short-chain fatty acids play in the gut. Short-chain fatty acids are metabolic products created by the gut bacteria when they process the dietary fiber that we eat. The three main fatty acids produced by the gut's microbes—acetic, propionic, and butyric acid—are either excreted or absorbed by the colon and used as a source of energy by the body's cells. By and large, butyric acid is the most important fuel for the cells lining the colon; this fatty acid is a primary energy source for colonic cells and has anti-carcinogenic as well as anti-inflammatory properties. The ratio of these fatty acids depends on the variety of gut bacteria as well as diet. In other words, different types of bacteria produce different short-chain fatty acids. Clostridial species produce propionic acid (PPA) in abundance, which, as you're about to learn, isn't a good thing if PPA passes into the bloodstream. In fact, the brain's exposure to PPA, as well as other molecules produced by certain gut bacteria, may be important keys to the autism puzzle.

THE PPA LINK

Simply put, the PPA produced by Clostridia is toxic to the brain, and its effects start in a gut overrun with these bacterial species. For starters, PPA increases gut permeability by weakening the tight junctions that hold the cells of the intestinal lining together. Without the right balance of gut microbes to keep this barrier intact, PPA can easily find its way to the other side, where it enters the bloodstream, trips the wire that turns on inflammation, and activates the immune system. PPA also affects cell-to-cell signaling, essentially crippling the way one cell can communicate with the next. PPA leads directly to compromised mitochondrial function, meaning it alters the brain's ability to use energy. It also increases oxidative stress, which in turn harms proteins, cell membranes, vital fats, and even DNA. And it depletes the brain of various molecules such as antioxidants, neurotransmitters, and omega-3 fats that the brain needs to run properly. Perhaps the most fascinating effect of PPA, how-ever, is what it has been shown to do in triggering symptoms of autism.

Dr. Derrick F. MacFabe is among the most prominent researchers in this area of medicine.[23] He's conducted some remarkable studies that have been published in our most respected journals. For more than a decade, MacFabe and his autism research group at Western Ontario University have been investigating how certain gut bacteria like Clostridia may interfere with brain development and function. When I spoke with him, he went as far as calling these bad bugs "infectious causes of autism." Let me highlight a few of his studies so you can see how he's drawn such a bold conclusion.

In one study, they fed pregnant rats and their offspring diets high in propionic acid.[24] By the time the pups were four to seven weeks old, their brains showed developmental changes similar to those seen in children with autism. MacFabe has also documented more immediate effects from PPA. When he and his team injected PPA into animals, they exhibited symptoms commonly associated with autism almost immediately. The rats developed repetitive behaviors and hyperactivity, and were seen turning in circles, moving backward, and losing their desire to socialize with other animals. They demonstrated increased anxiety and would "fixate on objects versus other animals"; they even had "favorite" objects. Incredibly, these effects happened *within two minutes* of administration of the PPA and lasted about 30 minutes, at which point the animals would revert to normal behavior.

MacFabe's group also documented increased inflammation in various cells in the brains of these animals. He told me that, for these reasons, he believes that autism may be an "acquired disorder involving altered PPA metabolism." It's one thing to read a scientific article detailing such an experiment. But it's another to see a video of these animals. Mac-Fabe recorded his experiment so the world can see the before and after. It's breathtaking, and you can see it for yourself on my website, where Dr. MacFabe has given me permission to post it.

Is there a way to counter the effects of PPA and reverse the damage? Dr. MacFabe has suggested the use of supplements containing important biomolecules that are often lacking in people with autism. These include L-carnitine, an amino acid critical to healthy brain function; omega-3 oils; and n-acetyl cysteine (NAC), the latter of which can enhance gluta-thione production. And we have plenty of evidence to show that individuals with autism are typically deficient in glutathione, a key antioxidant in the brain that helps control oxidative damage and inflammation.[25] In one 2013 study published in the *Journal of Neuroinflammation*, it was shown that rats pre-treated with NAC didn't experience the adverse changes in brain chemistry characteristic of autism once they were injected with PPA.[26] The NAC prevented changes in neurochemistry, inflammation, detoxification, and even damage to DNA that would have otherwise occurred with exposure to PPA. The authors concluded that if in fact PPA is determined to play a central role in autism, NAC "may be a promising therapeutic candidate for chemoprevention against PPA toxicity." They further cite another study that "proves the potential use-fulness of NAC for treating irritability and behavioural disturbance in children with autism."

In 2012, Stanford School of Medicine reported its own findings, showing that NAC supplementation lowered irritability and reduced repetitive behaviors in a group of children with autism. Many other such investigations over the past five years have shown promising results from treating children with autism with oral NAC and L-carnitine, but more research is needed.[27] I encourage anyone who is curious about trying these approaches to discuss them with your physician.

AUTISM AS A MITOCHONDRIAL DISORDER

If the story of autism were just about things like too much Clostridia and PPA, then eradicating the illness would be straightforward. But we know that autism is exceedingly complex and that the research is still in its early stages. I believe that more infectious agents will be identified that are associated with the development of the disorder. Clostridia are probably not the only species of bacteria that can overdevelop and overproduce molecules that are toxic to the brain if allowed into the bloodstream, stimulating the immune system and aggravating the neurological system. My guess is that future research will find other microbes that can be equally as harmful as Clostridia when it comes to brain function, and that could be implicated in the development of a disorder such as autism. It's interesting to note that autism incidence is extremely low in some developing populations such as Cambodia, a place far less hygienic than Western nations, where the diversity and number of microbes has been lessened through sanitation and dietary habits.

Authors of population-based studies have in fact coined a term, "Biome Depletion Theory," to describe the lack of microbes and even parasites in urban, post-industrial societies, where autism rates are relatively high. The lack of these organisms in Western cultures means that Western people's immune systems don't get to interact with these organisms and essentially build a stronger, smarter immune system to keep pathogenic microbes like Clostridia in check. This could be the reason why Western children's immune systems are overreacting, triggering an inflammatory response that manifests in autistic symptoms in vulnerable people.

To this end, I want to briefly highlight another set of studies that underscore the relevance of the microbiome in autism. In 2012, Caltech microbiologist Elaine Hsiao was among a team that conducted a fascinating experiment.[28] She based it on earlier evidence showing that women who get the flu during pregnancy double their risk of giving birth to a child with autism. She engineered mice by injecting pregnant females with a mock virus to gather pups with autism-like symptoms. The mock virus worked, and the mice gave birth to offspring that displayed classic signs of autism (in mice), such as obsessively licking themselves, burying marbles in their cages, and refusing to socialize with other mice. They also had leaky gut syndrome. Bingo. (To be clear, the virus doesn't necessarily have a severe effect on the mother-to-be; it triggers an infection-like immune response in her, which affects the growing baby.)

What Hsiao really wanted to find out was how the gut bacteria in these engineered mice influenced their behavior. She analyzed the mice's blood and discovered that the "autistic" mice contained a staggering 46 times more of a molecule like PPA, produced by gut bacteria and known to induce symptoms of autism when it's allowed to seep from the intestines into the blood.

Hsiao then laced the animals' food with B. *fragilis*, a probiotic that's been shown to treat GI problems in mice, and the results were jaw-dropping. Five weeks later, the leaky gut in "autistic" mice had sealed up, and the levels of the offending molecule in their blood had plummeted. Their behavior also changed, showing fewer symptoms of autism. The mice became less anxious and more social, and they stopped the repetitive behaviors.

To Hsiao's disappointment, however, the treated mice remained aloof when a new mouse was placed in their cage. This again points to the complexity of autism. The deficits seen in social interaction among many autistic kids are at the heart of the disorder. Obviously, B. *fragilis*, or any other single probiotic for that matter, is not a guaranteed treatment. But I have no doubt that future therapies for autism will include probiotics, some of which might work wonders on some symptoms of autism in some patients. I also have a hunch that in the future, we'll begin to view brain disorders like autism as mitochondrial diseases that have strong ties to the gut's tribes.

Throughout this book, I've made connections between conditions that you may not have initially thought were related to one another, such as the link between diabetes and dementia. I've also shared insights into common denominators in most brain ailments, notably inflammation. Even a disorder like autism has much in common with other brain disorders through the story of the mitochondria.[29] Neurological disorders as diverse as autism, schizophrenia, bipolar disorder, Parkinson's, and Alzheimer's have all been linked to mitochondrial glitches.[30] This is an important new clue to our understanding of these ailments, especially with regard to autism, because there are so many different degrees of severity on the spectrum.

In 2010, the *Journal of the American Medical Association* published an illuminating study that added yet another important piece to the autism puzzle.[31] Researchers at the University of California at Davis found that children with autism are far more likely to have shortfalls in their ability to produce cellular energy than are typically developing children, suggesting a strong link between autism and mitochondrial defects. Although previous studies had pointed to a connection between autism and mitochondrial dysfunction, this was the first to really establish the link and inspire others to further explore this area of research.

The UC Davis team recruited ten children aged two to five with autism and ten children of the same ages and from similar backgrounds who did not have autism. Taking blood samples from each child, the researchers focused on the mitochondria in immune cells, called lymphocytes, analyzing their metabolic pathways. They specifically sought to study the mitochondria of immune cells because previous studies had looked at mitochondria from muscle, but mitochondrial glitches are not always seen there. Muscle cells can generate a lot of their energy without relying on the mitochondria through a process called anaerobic glycolysis. Lymphocytes, on the other hand, as well as brain neurons, largely depend on the mitochondrial aerobic respiration for energy.

The results spoke for themselves: Children with autism showed signs of lowered mitochondrial activity, for their mitochondria consumed much less oxygen than mitochondria from the control children. Put another way, the mitochondria in the kids with autism couldn't keep up with the energy demands of their cells. As you can imagine, the brain is one of the biggest consumers of energy in the body, second only to the heart in its demands. The authors of the study hypothesized that deficiencies in the ability to fuel brain neurons could lead to some of the cognitive impairments associated with autism.

Remember, the mitochondria carry their own set of genetic instructions and are the cells' number one source of energy production. The researchers documented much higher levels of oxidative stress in the children with autism, as measured by higher levels of hydrogen peroxide with their mitochondria. What's more, two of the children with autism showed deletions in their mitochondrial DNA genes, a phenomenon not seen in the control children. The researchers concluded that all of these mitochondrial abnormalities measured in the mitochondria of children with autism suggest that oxidative stress in these vital organelles could be affecting autism's development and helping to determine its severity.

While these findings don't establish a cause for autism—the researchers don't know, for example, whether the mitochondria dysfunction initially occurred before or after these children were born—they certainly help refine the search for autism's origin. Dr. Isaac Pessah, director of the Center for Children's Environmental Health and Disease Prevention and a UC Davis MIND Institute researcher and professor of molecular biosciences at the UC Davis School of Veterinary Medicine, said, "The real challenge now is to try and understand the role of mitochondrial dysfunction in children with autism....Many environmental stressors can cause mitochondrial damage. Depending on when a child was exposed, maternally or neonatally, and how severe that exposure was, it might explain the range of the symptoms of autism."[32]

Statements like that are meaningful when you look at the bigger picture and consider the gut bacteria, too. Recall that in chapter 2 I mentioned that intestinal flora and mitochondria share a complex interplay and are like second and third sets of DNA in addition to our own nuclear DNA. Not only do the actions of gut bacteria support the health of the mitochondria, but when gut microbes are out of balance or dominated by pathogenic strains, they can inflict direct damage to the mitochondria through their toxic byproducts (e.g., PPA) or indirect damage through inflammatory pathways.

The notion that autism is characterized by unique patterns in both the microbiome and mitochondrial function will only continue to gain attention and traction in research circles. This is an exciting and burgeoning field, and I'm confident it will lead to better diagnostic tools and treatments. Although it may take years for us to tease apart the complex interplay among all the variables — the environmental factors, the mitochondrial and microbiome changes, as well as the actions of the immune and nervous systems — it shouldn't take years for us to appreciate the power of maintaining a healthy gut community. Whether or not gut microbes are a main player in the development of autism, or any neurological disorder, they are vital players in our complex physiology. And supporting them as best we can is perhaps the chief way we can influence our brain's health, and even our DNA.

TAKING CONTROL OF YOUR GENES

The idea that environment probably plays a large role in the development of autism, and that the roots of autism extend back into the very early days of a child's life, perhaps even before conception, is one that deserves more awareness. Even though genes encoded by DNA are essentially static (barring the occurrence of mutation), the expression of those genes can be highly dynamic in response to environmental influences. This field of study, called epigenetics, is now one of the hottest areas of research. We in the scientific community believe epigenetic forces affect us from our days in utero until the day we die. There are likely many windows during one's lifetime when we are sensitive to environmental impacts, and the time we spend in utero and during those early years of life represents a unique period of great vulnerability to influences that can change our biology and have major downstream effects, from autism to other neurological challenges in our youth and beyond. At the same time, the multitude of neural, immune, and hormonal actions that are controlled by the microbiome—and that in turn command our entire physiology—are susceptible to disruption and adaptation, especially by environmental changes.

Epigenetics, defined more technically, is the study of sections of your DNA (called "marks" or "markers") that essentially tell your genes when and how strongly to express themselves. Like conductors of an orchestra, these epigenetic marks control not only your health and longevity, but also how you pass your genes on to future generations. Indeed, the forces acting on the expression of your DNA today can be passed on to your future biological children, affecting how their genes behave in their lives and whether or not their children will face a higher risk for brain disorders like autism.

Many more years of research are needed to understand the relationship between gut bacteria and autism. I think the studies I highlighted in this chapter are promising, and could lead to new preventive measures and therapies that can help shift autism from being a debilitating disorder to a manageable condition. And best of all, these new therapies won't be pharmaceutical drugs that come with side effects. They will, for the most part, come from dietary choices and probiotic treatments to rebalance the microbiome. They will be lifestyle interventions that are highly accessible and economical for everyone.

As we come to the end of part I and move into part II, where I describe the environmental factors in changing the microbiome, I want you to keep in mind that our day-to-day lifestyle choices have a big effect on our biology and even the activity of our genes. What's empowering about this is that we can change our health's destiny, as well as the destiny of our children's health, if we make the right choices. Now that we have evidence to suggest that food, stress, exercise, sleep—and the state of our microbiome—affect which of our genes are activated and which remain suppressed, we can take some degree of control in all of these realms. To be sure, we may never be able to totally eradicate the possibility of autism or another brain disorder, but we can most certainly do our best to reduce the chances. And now that we know that the gut bacteria factor in somewhere, harnessing the microbiome for the benefit of the brain becomes key. What also becomes key is knowing how a good microbiome can go bad. Hence the purpose of part II.

TROUBLE IN BUGVILLE

Is your headache medicine toxic to your gut bacteria? Can regular and diet soda assassinate healthy microbial tribes? Do foods made from genetically modified organisms (GMOs) foment trouble in the body?

Now that you've gotten a panoramic view of the microbiome, it's time to turn to the common exposures that can corrupt it. These include not only dietary factors and drugs, but also chemicals in the environment, the water we drink, the clothes we buy, and the personal care products we use. Although it seems that virtually anything can affect the microbiome, in this part of the book I focus on the biggest culprits over which you have some control. None of us can live in a bubble or avoid all exposure to substances that threaten our microbiome. But it pays to be aware of the most villainous ones. Knowledge, after all, is power. With the lessons learned in part II, you'll be fully prepared to execute my recommendations outlined in part III.

CHAPTER 6

Punched in the Gut

The Truth about Fructose and Gluten

WHEN PEOPLE ASK ME TO list all the things that can destroy a healthy adult microbiome, I explain that it all comes down to what you're exposed to and what you put into your mouth. Obviously, by the time you've grown up, you've already had the cards either stacked in your favor or not, depending on how you came into this world and what your early life was like. Although there's nothing you can do to reverse your personal history, you can take charge—starting today—to change the state of your gut and the fate of your brain. And it starts with diet.

Anyone who has read *Grain Brain* knows my take on the power of diet to effect positive change in human health and the course of disease. But my perspective isn't just my own, and it's far from a casual opinion based on anecdotal evidence. It's backed by rigorous science, some of which has just come out and is truly spectacular. And what the latest science is showing is that changes in human nutrition are not just responsible for so many of our common maladies; they directly correlate with changes in the gut bacteria.

In a beautifully written and well-cited review of what we know so far about the complex diet–gut–microbes–health equation, Canadian researchers stated the following: "Overall, dietary changes could explain 57% of the total structural variation in gut microbiota whereas changes in genetics accounted for no more than 12%. This indicates that diet has a dominating role in shaping gut microbiota and changing key populations may transform healthy gut microbiota into a disease-inducing entity."[1]

Let me repeat: *Diet has the dominant role in shaping gut microbiota, and changing key populations may transform healthy gut microbiota into a disease-inducing entity.* If there's only one fact you take away from this book, that sentence is it. Dr. Alessio Fasano of Harvard, one of the leading authorities on the gut-brain connection, whom I introduced at the beginning of the book, has echoed this same sentiment. In fact, he shared with me during a conference that while antibiotics and method of birth are important factors in the development and maintenance of a healthy microbiome, dietary choices are far and away the most crucial factor.

So what kind of diet makes for an optimal microbiome? I'll get to all of those details in chapter 9. For now, let's focus on the top two ingredients to avoid when it comes to preserving the health, balance, and function of your belly bugs.

FRUCTOSE

As I've mentioned, fructose has become one of the most common sources of calories in the Western diet. Fructose is naturally found in fruit, but that's not where we're getting it from; most of the fructose we consume is from manufactured sources. Our caveman ancestors did eat fruit, but only during certain times of the year when it was available; our bodies haven't yet evolved to healthily manage the prodigious amounts of fructose we consume today. Natural whole fruit has relatively little sugar when compared to, say, a can of regular soda or concentrated juice. A medium-size apple contains a little over 70 calories from sugar in a fiber-rich blend; conversely, a 12-ounce can of regular soda contains twice that—140 calories of sugar. A 12-ounce glass of apple juice (no pulp) is about equal with the soda, clocking in at the same number of sugar calories. Your body wouldn't know the difference whether the sugar came from a juiced batch of apples or a soda factory.

Of all naturally occurring carbohydrates, fructose is the sweetest. No wonder we love it so much. But, contrary to what you might think, it doesn't have a high glycemic index. In fact, it has the lowest GI of all the natural sugars because the liver metabolizes most of the fructose, so it has no immediate effect on our blood-sugar and insulin levels. This is quite unlike table sugar or high-fructose corn syrup, whose glucose ends up in general circulation and raises blood-sugar levels.

That fact doesn't let fructose off the hook, so to speak. Fructose has long-term effects when it's consumed in large quantities from unnatural sources. Numerous studies show that fructose is associated with impaired glucose tolerance, insulin resistance, high blood fats, and hypertension. It's a huge burden to the liver, which is forced to expend so much energy converting fructose into other molecules that it risks not having enough left for all of its other functions. One of the fallouts of this energy depletion is the production of uric acid, a consequence linked to high blood pressure, gout, and kidney stones. Moreover, because fructose doesn't trigger the production of insulin and leptin, two hormones key to regulating metabolism, diets high in fructose often lead to obesity and its metabolic repercussions. I should add that the fiber in fruits and vegetables slows down absorption of fructose into the bloodstream. Conversely, high-fructose corn syrup and crystalline fructose disrupt liver metabolism, which, along with excess glucose, spikes blood-sugar levels and exhausts the pancreas. To clarify, high-fructose corn syrup (HFCS) actually doesn't come from fruit; as its name implies, it's a sweetener made from corn syrup. Specifically, corn starch is processed to yield a type of glucose that can be further processed with enzymes to produce a clear substance that's high in fructose and has a longer shelf life than regular table sugar. HFCS ends up being a mixture of about half fructose and half glucose, the latter of which raises blood-sugar levels.

As I mentioned in chapter 4, new research shows that obesity might be a reflection of the changes in the microbiome *brought on by fructose exposure.* Such changes may have served us in Paleolithic times to increase our production of fat in late summer when fruit ripened and fructose was consumed. Excess fat helped us survive through the winter when food was scarce, but this mechanism has become maladaptive in our modern world, where fructose is abundant.

Interestingly enough, the fact that our gut bacteria are affected by the sugar we consume has just recently been revealed from studies done on artificial sweeteners. The human body cannot digest artificial sweeteners, which is why they have no calories. But they still must pass through the gastrointestinal tract. For a long time we assumed that artificial sweeteners were, for the most part, inert ingredients in terms of affecting our physiology. Far from it. In 2014, a bombshell paper that I briefly mentioned in chapter 4 was published in *Nature.*[2]

Professor Eran Segal, a computational biologist at the Weizmann Institute of Science in Israel, led his team in a series of experiments to answer one question: Do artificial sweeteners affect healthy gut bacteria? Segal and his colleagues started by adding the fake sugars saccharin, sucralose, or aspartame to the drinking water of different groups of mice. They gave other mouse groups the real sugars glucose or sucrose (a combination of glucose and fructose) in their water. Their control group drank plain, unsweetened water. Eleven weeks later, the mice that received the artificial sweeteners exhibited signs that they weren't able to process real sugar well, as measured by higher levels of glucose intolerance compared with the others. To see whether gut bacteria had anything to do with the link between drinking fake sugar and developing glucose intolerance, the researchers gave the mice antibiotics for four weeks to essentially exterminate their gut bacteria. Lo and behold, after the annihilation all the mouse groups were able to metabolize sugar equally well.

Next, the researchers transplanted gut bacteria from mice that had consumed saccharin into germ-free mice with no gut bacteria of their own. Within just six days, the tainted mice had lost some of their ability to process sugar. The genetic analyses of the gut colonies spoke for themselves, revealing a shift in composition of the gut bacteria upon exposure to the artificial sweetener. Some types of bacteria became more abundant, while others diminished.

Research is now underway on humans, and so far preliminary results indeed show that artificial sugar isn't what it's long been cracked up to be — a safe and healthier alternative to real sugar. Studies are emerging that show that gut bacteria of people who regularly consume artificial sweeteners look different from gut bacteria of people who do not. Correlations have also been found between those who use artificial sweeteners and those who weigh more and have higher fasting blood sugar, a condition we know leads to many negative health effects. Moreover, in another watershed study published in 2013, French researchers had followed more than 66,000 women since 1993 and found that the risk for developing diabetes was *more than double* for those who drank artificially sweetened drinks than it was for women who consumed sugar-sweetened beverages.[3] Take a look (but don't interpret this data to mean you can drink sugar-sweetened drinks):

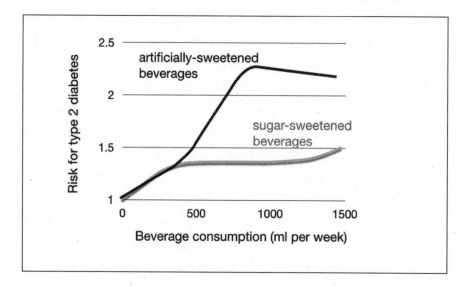

Now, let me bring this conversation back to fructose. The average American eats 80 grams of fructose each day, often in the processed form of high-fructose corn syrup. It's impossible for all of that to get absorbed from the gut into the bloodstream. Gut bugs love processed fructose as much as the average human does, maybe more so, and they feast on any excess in the gut. The fructose is rapidly fermented by the gut bacteria, resulting in byproducts like those short-chain fatty acids we discussed in chapter 5, as well as a potpourri of gases, including methane, hydrogen, carbon dioxide, and hydrogen sulfide. As you can imagine, fermenting gases build up and can cause bloating, discomfort, or abdominal pain. Excess fructose in the gut also pulls excess water with it, which can have a laxative effect. Adding insult to injury, those short-chain fatty acids also draw more water to the bowel.

Contrary to what you might think, methane gas is not inert. A number of experiments have shown that excess methane in the large intestine is biologically active. It can disrupt the actions of the colon and impede digestion and the movement of stool, leading to abdominal pain and constipation.

Processed fructose's disturbing effects don't end there; it's also been linked to rapid liver damage—*even without weight gain*. In a study published in 2013 in the *American Journal of Clinical Nutrition*, researchers showed that high fructose can cause bacteria to exit the intestines, go into the bloodstream, and damage the liver.[4] In the words of the study's lead author, Dr. Kylie Kavanagh of Wake Forest Baptist Medical Center, "It appears that something about the high fructose levels was causing the intestines to be less protective than normal, and consequently allowing the bacteria to leak out at a 30 percent higher rate." The study based its conclusions on animal models (monkeys), but it likely reflects what goes on in the human gut and helps explain how thin people who consume lots of processed fructose yet remain lean can still suffer from metabolic dysfunction and liver disease. More human studies are under way.

So the next time you're tempted to guzzle a regular or diet soda, or chow down on a food product loaded with high-fructose corn syrup, I hope you think again. In part III, I'll give you some tips for sweetening up your foods without disrupting your gut bugs.

GLUTEN

I saved the best (or worst, depending on how you look at it) for last. I wrote extensively about gluten in *Grain Brain*, calling the protein found in wheat, barley, and rye among the most inflammatory ingredients of the modern era. I argued that while a small percentage of the population is highly sensitive to gluten and suffers from celiac disease, it's possible for virtually *everyone* to have a negative, albeit undetected, reaction. Gluten sensitivity—with or without the presence of celiac—increases the production of inflammatory cytokines, which are pivotal players in neurodegenerative conditions. And as I've been implying, the brain is among the most susceptible organs to the deleterious effects of inflammation.

I call gluten a "silent germ" because it can inflict lasting damage without your knowing it. While its effects might start with unexplained headaches and feeling anxious, or "wired and tired," they can worsen to more dire disorders such as depression and dementia. Gluten is everywhere today, despite the gluten-free movement taking place even among food manufacturers. It lurks in everything from wheat products to ice cream to hand cream. It's even used as an additive in seemingly "healthy," wheat-free products. I can't even begin to list the number of studies that have confirmed the irrefutable connection between gluten sensitivity and neurological dysfunction. Even people who are not clinically sensitive to gluten (they test negative and don't appear to have issues digesting the protein) can suffer problems.

I see the effects of gluten every day in my practice. My patients often reach me only after they've been to a slew of other doctors and have "tried everything." Whether they're suffering from headaches or migraines, anxiety, ADHD, depression, memory problems, MS, ALS, autism, or just some odd set of neurological symptoms with no definite label, one of the first things I do is prescribe the total elimination of gluten from their diets. And I continue to be astounded by the results. To be clear, I'm not saying that gluten is specifically playing a causal role in a disease like ALS, but when we see scientific data demonstrating profound gut permeability in this disorder, it makes sense to do everything you can to reduce this process. And eliminating gluten is an important first step.

Gluten is made up of two main groups of proteins, the *glutenins* and the *gliadins*. You can be sensitive to either of these proteins or to one of the twelve different, smaller units that make up gliadin. A reaction to any of these could lead to inflammation.

Even since I wrote *Grain Brain*, new research has come to light about the damaging effects of gluten on the microbiome. Indeed, it's quite possible that the entire cascade of adverse effects that takes place when the body is exposed to gluten starts with a change in the microbiome—ground zero. Before I explain this cascade, let me remind you of a few important facts. Some of this will be familiar to you, but it's important to understand this message, especially as it relates to gluten.

Gluten's "sticky" attribute interferes with the breakdown and absorption of nutrients, which leads to poorly digested food that can then sound the alarm in the immune system, eventually resulting in an assault on the lining of the small intestine. Those who experience symptoms of gluten sensitivity complain of abdominal pain, nausea, diarrhea, constipation, and intestinal distress. Many people, however, don't experience these blatant signs of gastrointestinal trouble, yet they could be experiencing a silent attack elsewhere in their body, such as in their nervous system.

Once the alarm has sounded, the immune system sends out inflammatory chemicals in a bid to get things under control and neutralize the effects of the enemies. This process can damage tissues, leaving the walls of the intestine compromised, a condition that you know by now is called "leaky gut." According to Harvard's Dr. Alessio Fasano, exposure to the gliadin protein in particular increases gut permeability *in all of us*.[5] That's right, all humans have some degree of gluten sensitivity. Once you have a leaky gut, you're highly susceptible to other food sensitivities in the future. You're also vulnerable to the impact of LPS making its way into the bloodstream. Lipopolysaccharide, or LPS as you'll recall, is a structural component of many microbial cells in the gut. If LPS gets past those tight junctions, it increases systemic inflammation and irritates the immune system—a double strike that puts you at risk for myriad brain ailments, autoimmune disease, and cancer.

The hallmark of gluten sensitivity is elevated levels of antibodies against the gliadin component of gluten, which turn on specific genes in certain immune cells and trigger the release of the brain-assaulting inflammatory cytokine chemicals. This process has been described in the medical literature for decades. Anti-gliadin antibodies also appear to cross-react with certain brain proteins. A study published in 2007 in the *Journal of Immunology* found that anti-gliadin antibodies bind to neuronal synapsin I, a neuronal protein. In their conclusions, the study's authors said that this may explain why gliadin contributes to "neurologic complications such as neuropathy, ataxia, seizures, and neurobehavioral changes."[6]

Research has also shown that the immune system's reaction to gluten does more than just push the button on inflammation. Dr. Fasano's research reveals that the same mechanism by which gluten increases inflammation and gut permeability also leads to a breakdown of the blood-brain barrier itself, paving the way for the production of yet more brain-crushing inflammatory chemicals.[7, 8] I test all of my patients who have unexplained neurological disorders for gluten sensitivity. In fact, the same company—Cyrex Labs—that does the blood screening tests for LPS also performs high-tech tests for gluten sensitivity (go to www .DrPerlmutter.com/Resources for more about these important tests).

Now, let's circle back to the microbiome. As I described in chapter 5, alterations in the composition of short-chain fatty acids, which play a critical role in maintaining the intestinal lining, are a flagrant signal that the composition of the gut bacteria has shifted (remember that these acids are produced by gut bacteria; different types of gut bacteria produce different types of these fatty acids). The latest evidence reveals that among those who exhibit the most adverse changes in these short-chain fatty acids, celiac patients win the award, reflecting a consequence of altered gut bacteria.[9] It appears to work both ways, too; alterations of the microbiota are now recognized as playing an active role in the pathogenesis of celiac disease. Said another way, an imbalanced microbial community in the gut can stoke and intensify celiac disease just as the presence of the disorder incites changes in the gut bacteria. And this is relevant because celiac disease is associated with a host of neurological complications from epilepsy to dementia.

Let's not forget the other facts of the matter: Children born by C-section and those who've taken lots of antibiotics are at a much higher risk for developing celiac disease, and this heightened risk is a direct function of the quality of the developing microbiome and how many insults it has weathered. And children at risk for celiac disease have been well described in the literature as having notably fewer Bacteroidetes, the type of bacteria associated with better health.[10] This may be why children and adults in Western cultures have a higher risk for inflammatory and autoimmune conditions compared to people living in areas of the world where microbiomes are rife with Bacteroidetes.

The most compelling evidence we have to date for going gluten-free to preserve health and brain function comes from the Mayo Clinic. In 2013, a team of doctors and researchers there finally showed how dietary gluten might cause type 1 diabetes. Although studies have long shown a connection between the ingestion of gluten and the development of type 1 diabetes, this was the first study to uncover the real mechanism. In the study, the researchers fed non-obese mice prone to type 1 diabetes either a gluten-free diet or one that contained gluten. The gluten-free mice lucked out; their diet protected them from type 1 diabetes. When the researchers added gluten back into the diets of these healthy mice, it reversed the protective effect the gluten-free diet had provided. The researchers also noted a measurable impact of the gluten on the bacterial flora of the mice, leading the scientists to conclude that "the presence of gluten is directly responsible for the pro-diabetogenic effects of diets and it determines the gut microflora. Our novel study thus suggests that dietary gluten could modulate the incidence of [type 1 diabetes] by changing the gut microbiome."[11] (For the record, type 1 diabetes is an autoimmune disorder that affects a very small number of people, compared to type 2 diabetes.)

This new study followed closely in the wake of another study published in the same journal, the *Public Library of Science*, which found that the alcohol-soluble portion of gluten, the gliadin, promotes weight gain and pancreatic beta cell hyperactivity, a potential contributor to type 2 diabetes and a precursor to type 1 diabetes.[12] These conditions, as you know, are huge risk factors for brain disease. Given the increasingly dense body of research, the time has come to recognize that many of the most common ailments that afflict us today are a direct result of the consumption of popular foods such as wheat.

I realize that much has been written about whether or not the gluten-free craze is health or hype. For those of you who test negative to gluten sensitivity or who have never had problems with gluten and love your pancakes and pizza, let me share the following: Research shows that modern wheat is capable of producing more than 23,000 different proteins, any one of which could trigger a potentially damaging inflammatory response.[13] While we know the harmful effects that gluten can have, I predict that future research will reveal more injurious proteins that travel with gluten in modern grains and that have equally, if not more, deleterious effects on the body and brain.

Going gluten-free today does come with challenges. Although there's a huge market now for gluten-free products, the bottom line is they are just that—products, and they can be just as junky and nutrient-poor as processed products that don't come with a "gluten-free" claim. Many are made with refined, gluten-free grains that are low in fiber, vitamins, and other nutrients. That's why it's crucial to pay attention to ingredients and choose gluten-free foods that are authentic in their nutrition and wholesomeness. I'll help you do that in part III.

I like to tell patients that cleaning up their diet to nix gluten and manufactured fructose, while limiting natural fructose from real fruit, is step 1 in preserving the health and function of their microbiome and brain. Step 2, as you're about to read, is managing exposures to chemicals and drugs that can also have health implications—the focus of this next chapter.

CHAPTER 7

Bust a Gut

Common Exposures That Make a Good Microbiome Go Bad

Now that we've squared away the top dietary hazards to a healthy microbiome, let's get a little closer to the science of what else threatens your gut's community from the perspective of drugs and environmental chemicals. I outline the worst offenders below. Some of this information reiterates concepts we've already explored, while giving you additional data to empower the new choices you're going to make in your life going forward.

ANTIBIOTICS

I vividly remember when I was five years old and my father suddenly became weak. At that time he was a busy neurosurgeon, covering five or six hospitals while at the same time being Dad for his five children (I am the youngest). Dad was very driven, as you can imagine, but suddenly he began experiencing fevers and overwhelming fatigue. He consulted several of his colleagues and ultimately was diagnosed with subacute bacterial endocarditis, an infection of the heart caused by the organism *Streptococcus viridans*. Dad received penicillin intravenously for three months. It was administered at home, and I can recall watching him read his medical journals with the IV bag hanging next to his bed. Had it not been for penicillin, this infection would have undoubtedly proven fatal. So I understand, loud and clear, the importance and effectiveness of antibiotics. Nonetheless, I can't help but wonder about the changes that his microbiome endured during this treatment, and how that may have played a role in his current situation with Alzheimer's disease.

I can't talk about the role of antibiotics in the course of human health without paying tribute to them. I know plenty of friends, family members, and colleagues who would not be with us today had it not been for antibiotics. Serious diseases that once killed millions of people each year can easily be treated today thanks to antibiotics. The discovery of antibiotics ("against life") in the early part of the 20th century has been one of our most significant medical achievements.

In 1928, British scientist Alexander Fleming discovered, almost by accident, a naturally growing substance — a fungus — that could kill certain bacteria. He was cultivating the common *Staphylococcus aureus* bacteria when he noted that a mold in the same dish was annihilating his colony. He named the mold *Penicillium,* and he and others would go on to conduct numerous experiments using penicillin to destroy infectious bacteria. Eventually, researchers in Europe and the U.S. began testing penicillin in animals and then humans. In 1941, even low levels of penicillin were found to cure very serious infections and save many lives. In 1945, Alexander Fleming won the Nobel Prize in Physiology and Medicine.

Anne Miller was the first person to benefit from the life-saving drug in the U.S. In 1942, she was a 33-year-old nurse who had suffered a miscarriage. She came down with a very serious illness called childbirth fever, technically known as puerperal sepsis, caused by a severe streptococcal infection in the body. Anne was critically ill for a month with high fevers and delirium. Her doctor was able to get his hands on one of the first batches of penicillin, even though it wasn't commercially available yet. The drug was shipped by aircraft and delivered to state troopers in Connecticut, who handed the vial over to doctors at Yale–New Haven Hospital where Anne lay on her near-deathbed.

Within hours of administering the drug—1 teaspoonful containing 5.5 grams of penicillin—Anne's health turned around quickly. The fever abated, the delirium broke, her appetite returned, and within a month she was fully recovered. The drug was so coveted and supplies were so low that Anne's urine was saved so it could be filtered for remnants of the drug to be purified and used again. Anne was back at Yale in 1992 for the fiftieth anniversary of this landmark event. She was then in her eighties and would live until age ninety. Had it not been for penicillin, she would have met her death more than half a century sooner.

Of course, antibiotics aren't magic bullets that can eradicate every infection. When used at the right time, however, they can cure many serious and life-threatening illnesses. They have revolutionized medicine, but the pendulum has swung far from those days when antibiotics were rarely available. Today they are everywhere and far too often overused.

Four out of five Americans take an antibiotic every year, according to the CDC.[1] About 258 million courses of antibiotics were prescribed in 2010 in the U.S. for a population of 309 million people. Antibiotics constitute the majority of prescriptions for children under ten years old. Extravagant use of antibiotics, especially for viral illnesses, which are not helped by these drugs (e.g., colds, flus), has led to the proliferation of antibiotic-resistant strains of bad pathogens that current antibiotics cannot touch. The World Health Organization (WHO) has stated: "Without urgent action we are heading for a post-antibiotic era, in which common infections and minor injuries can once again kill."[2] The organization has called antibiotic resistance one of the "top health challenges facing the 21st century."

Alexander Fleming himself warned us about these potential consequences back in 1945 during his Nobel Prize lecture, when he said, "The time may come when penicillin can be bought by anyone in the shops. Then there is the danger that the ignorant man may easily underdose himself and, by exposing his microbes to non-lethal quantities of the drug, make them resistant."[3] (When using antibiotics, "underdosing"— taking too little or failing to complete a prescribed round—can be just as problematic as over-using antibiotics in general. Both practices lead to resistant, rogue strains.) It was only three years later that mutant staphylococcus strains, impervious to penicillin, emerged. Today, methicillin-resistant *Staphylococcus aureus* (MRSA) infection is caused by a wicked strain of staph bacteria that cannot be treated by most of the common antibiotics. MRSA has become a huge threat here in the U.S., killing people with weak immune systems and sending young, otherwise healthy people to hospitals for treatment. Overall, two million Americans suffer drug-resistant infections annually, and 23,000 of them die.[4] Tuberculosis is also making a comeback, thanks to virulent strains of *Mycobacterium tuberculosis* that ravage the lungs.

Antibiotics are also used extensively in agriculture and farming, and this is contributing to the problem of resistance. They are used to treat infection as well as to make animals grow larger and mature earlier. Animal lab studies reveal that big changes occur quickly (as little as two weeks) in livestock's microbiomes when they receive antibiotics—changes that promote obesity thanks to the kinds of bacteria left in the wake of the antibiotic exposure (more on this shortly), and that cause a significant increase in antibiotic resistance. These antibiotics eventually find their way into meats, poultry, and dairy products, and this has raised concerns about their lingering effects in the human body. Antibiotics are endocrine-disrupters, and constant exposure to these drugs in our food supply mimics and confuses sex hormones in the body. They may also tinker with our metabolism, fueling obesity. And this metabolic tinkering may be happening through the antibiotics' direct effects in the body as well as through the gut bacteria.

There's a lot of debate today about whether the childhood obesity epidemic can partly be blamed on the cumulative effects these drugs have had on children's vulnerable, developing bodies. Unfortunately, there are many legal and political loopholes in legislative efforts to reduce antibiotics in the food supply.

Key to our discussion is, of course, the damaging effects of these drugs on the human microbiome. For example, the mechanism by which antibiotics make cattle—and probably humans—heavier is through changes in the microbiome. Recall in chapter 4 how I described the difference between the types of gut bacteria that lead to more fat storage and weight gain and the types that prevent obesity. Firmicutes can harvest more energy from food, thereby increasing the risk of the body absorbing more calories and gaining weight. The guts of obese humans are routinely found to be dominated by Firmicutes, as opposed to Bacteroidetes, which are predominant in the guts of lean individuals. What happens when an animal, be it a cow or human, takes antibiotics is that the body's microbiome is instantly changed in diversity and composition as the antibiotics immediately wipe out certain strains, leaving others to flourish. And unfortunately, antibiotics can create a massive imbalance whereby the gut is rife with obesity-promoting bacteria. Dr. Martin Blaser of New York University is among the researchers who speculate that antibiotic usage contributes to obesity. In fact, his studies have looked at the effects of antibiotics on one particular infamous strain of bacteria that I've already mentioned: *H. pylori*, a popular target of doctors for patients who suffer from peptic ulcers. While it's been shown to increase the risk for peptic ulcers and gastric cancer, it's a common member of the human gut microbial community.

In one of Dr. Blaser's studies, done in 2011, he examined U.S. veterans who were undergoing tests to look closely at the upper gastrointestinal tract.[5] Of the ninety-two veterans, 38 tested negative for *H. pylori*, 44 tested positive, and 10 were indeterminate. Twenty-three of the men with *H. pylori* were given antibiotics, which wiped out the bacteria in all of the men except for two. And about those twenty-one veterans who eradicated *H. pylori* through antibiotics, guess what: They gained the most weight. Their BMIs increased by about 5 percent, plus or minus 2 percent. The other vets had no weight change. What's more, their levels of the appetite-stimulating hormone ghrelin increased sixfold after a meal, indicating that they weren't feeling full yet from their meals and could eat more. High levels of ghrelin are also known to increase abdominal fat. So the facts of antibiotics as growth promoters make sense when you put it all together. They most definitely help pack on the pounds in livestock. And they are helping us pack on the pounds, too, when antibiotics are used or consumed through foods.

As you can see in the graph below, the U.S. leads the way in terms of antibiotic use in meat produced.[6]

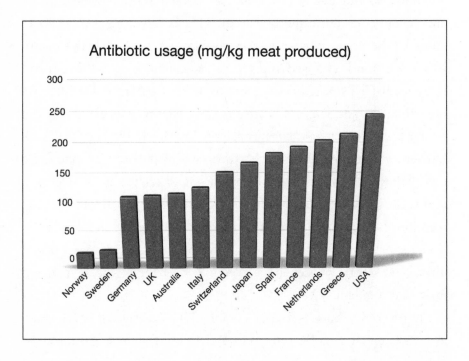

In 2011, U.S. drug makers sold nearly 30 million pounds of antibiotics for livestock, the largest amount yet recorded, representing 80 percent of all antibiotics sales that year.[7]

The FDA only began testing meat and poultry for antibiotic-resistant bacteria in 1996, and the politics of policing antibiotic use is, sadly, an impediment for real and transparent oversight. Dr. David Kessler, a former FDA commissioner and bestselling author of *The End of Overeating*, stated the facts well when he wrote an op-ed for the *New York Times* in 2013: "Why are lawmakers so reluctant to find out how 80 percent of our antibiotics are used? We cannot avoid tough questions because we're afraid of the answers. Lawmakers must let the public know how the drugs they need to stay well are being used to produce cheaper meat."[8]

Although it may take a painfully long time for tighter restrictions and regulations to be put into place regarding antibiotic use in the food supply, I'm happy to see change already occurring at the level of the CDC, WHO, and American Medical Association regarding prescribed antibiotics for infections. These institutions have already issued multiple warnings that doctors are now listening to. This has led to greater awareness about which kinds of infections truly need antibiotics and which would be best left alone for the body to take care of naturally. The goal is to curtail the usage of antibiotics unless they are absolutely necessary. Just in the last couple of years, for example, pediatricians have been urged to not have that knee-jerk response to parents asking for antibiotics to treat their child's ear or throat infection. That's the kind of change I'd like to see.

According to the *Journal of the American Medical Association*, these infections can usually be treated without antibiotics:[9]

- Common cold

- Influenza (flu)

- Most coughs and bronchitis

- Many ear infections

- Many skin rashes

In 2004, an exceedingly unnerving study published in the *Journal of the American Medical Association* brought home for me the impact of antibiotics when researchers demonstrated their potential to significantly increase one's risk for cancer.[10] University of Washington researchers looked at 2,266 women older than 19 with primary invasive breast cancer (breast cancer that has the potential to spread from the breast to other parts of the body) and compared them to 7,953 randomly selected female controls. The study was designed to determine whether there was an increased risk of breast cancer in women who'd taken antibiotics (all types). Lo and behold, the researchers found a clear link between the number of days of antibiotic use and an increased risk of breast cancer. In those individuals who'd taken the most antibiotics, the risk of breast cancer was *doubled*. The results also showed a significant correlation between antibiotic use and terminal breast cancer. The authors stated: "Use of antibiotics is associated with increased risk of incident and fatal breast cancer." They concluded, "Although further studies are needed, these findings reinforce the need for prudent long-term use of antibiotics."

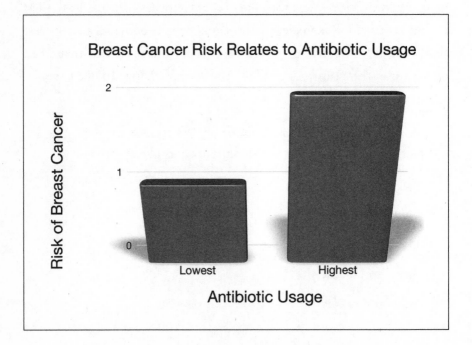

To be clear, this study did not indicate that antibiotics cause breast cancer. But, given what we know about how these potent drugs alter the gut bacteria as well as microbes' role in immunity, detoxification, and inflammation, studies like this should at least raise our suspicions. I expect more high-profile studies to emerge in the next decade showing a powerful relationship between the state of the gut's microbiome and the risk of certain cancers, including cancers of the brain and nervous system.

Dr. Robert F. Schwabe is one investigator leading the charge in this area. A research physician at Columbia University's Department of Medicine, Dr. Schwabe wrote a convincing article in 2013, published in a specialty journal for *Nature*, that outlined the means by which the condition of the microbiome can either promote or prevent cancerous growths.[11] In his concluding thoughts, he emphasizes the value in turning our attention to the study of the microbiome in hopes of finding new therapies for the prevention and treatment of cancer, calling the microbiome "the next frontier of medical research."

I used the example of cancer to further accuse antibiotics of ruining an important collaborator in our health, but I actually could just as easily have talked about exposure to antibiotics and a heightened risk of ADHD, asthma, being overweight, and diabetes — all of which significantly increase risk for dementia, depression, suicide, and anxiety. By now you can guess the thread tying all of these conditions together: inflammation. And if you take one more step back from the inflammatory process, you'll find yourself thinking about your gut's microbiota.

Several times a week my phone rings at my office with patients asking me to "call something in" because they've got a cold. I always explain that it's inappropriate. And when they specifically request a Zithromax Z-Pak, one of the most commonly prescribed antibiotics for upper respiratory infections, I give them the facts: Data from large groups of patients shows that use of this antibiotic significantly increases the risk of a heart-related death, because one of the potential side effects of the drug is heart arrhythmias.[12] In fact, in one of the studies examining this link, researchers at the University of South Carolina Medical School estimated that half of the 40 million prescriptions filled for this antibiotic in 2011 were unnecessary and may have caused 4,560 deaths.[13] I also like to tell patients who ask for antibiotics that if they don't take an antibiotic their cold will probably last about a week, but if they do take one, it'll only last seven days. I'm not sure they always get the joke. It seems as if all the news related to the dangers of antibiotic overuse is falling on deaf ears. This isn't about just you or me. It's about all of us.

The next time you think you or your child needs an antibiotic, I encourage you to weigh the pros and cons. It goes without saying that if it's an infection that can only be cured with antibiotics, by all means use them wisely and exactly as the doctor prescribes (see page 212 for more details about supplementing with probiotics during the antibiotic course). But if it's an infection that cannot be helped by antibiotics, consider how much you're "saving" in terms of the microbiome. This is especially true when it comes to children, who are uniquely vulnerable. It's recently been shown, for instance, that the vast majority of kids would recover from an ear infection within a few days if given medication only to relieve pain or fevers. In a 2010 study published in the *Journal of the American Medical Association*, a group of pediatricians sounded the alarm on the overuse of antibiotics for these common infections that are often caused by viruses.[14] The doctors noted that the risk of side effects from taking antibiotics outweighs the benefits, which are nil in most cases. A round of antibiotics, or multiple rounds, will increase children's risk for a variety of health challenges stemming from the disrupted gut bacteria—from asthma and obesity in their youth to dementia later in life. It's all connected. The gut bacteria create those enduring links.

NOTE TO PEOPLE WHO TAKE ANTIBIOTICS BEFORE GOING TO THE DENTIST

Many of my older patients who've had total hip or knee replacements tell me that they always take antibiotics as a prophylactic prior to visiting the dentist. The practice has been going on for so long that people just generally accept that this makes sense. But current science tells us otherwise: The latest research indicates that there is absolutely no benefit in taking antibiotics for dental procedures if you have a total hip or knee prosthesis. In the words of one recent study's conclusion: "Dental procedures were not risk factors for subsequent total hip or knee infection. The use of antibiotic prophylaxis prior to dental procedures did not decrease the risk of subsequent total hip or knee infection."[15]

That said, there are some individuals who should consider prophylactic antibiotics prior to dental procedures, specifically procedures that entail dental or gum surgery. But only a small number of people land in this category, including people with the following:

- Prior infective endocarditis

- Prosthetic cardiac valves

- Unrepaired cyanotic congenital heart defects, including palliative shunts and conduits

- Congenital heart defects completely repaired with prosthetic material or a device, whether placed by surgery or by catheter intervention, during the first 6 months after the procedure

- Repaired congenital defects with residual defects at the site or adjacent to the site of a prosthetic patch or prosthetic device

- Cardiac transplants and development of cardiac valvulopathy

And if you don't know what these things are, then you don't qualify to need prophylactic antibiotics before having oral surgery.

THE PILL

Millions of women of childbearing age take birth control. Since the Pill, as it's known, was first developed in the 1960s, it has been hailed as one of the cornerstones of the feminist movement. But birth control pills are, after all, synthetic hormones that have immediate biological effects on the human body, and they inevitably take a toll on the microbial community. Although virtually all medicines have some impact on the microbiome, drugs like the Pill, that are taken daily and often long-term, are the most insidious. Among the many outcomes of long-term use (more than five years) are:

- Decreased thyroid hormone and available testosterone in circulation

- Increased insulin resistance, oxidative stress, and markers of inflammation

- Depletion of certain vitamins, minerals, and antioxidants

Given all I've already explained about gut bacteria's role in metabolism, immunology, neurology, and even endocrinology, it's no wonder that they'd be impacted by "the naughty little pill," a term Manhattan psychiatrist Dr. Kelly Brogan uses to describe the Pill to her patients. It's also no wonder that among the most common side effects noted in using the Pill are mood and anxiety disorders. One of the vitamins depleted by the Pill is B6, which is a cofactor for the production of serotonin and GABA—two key molecules in brain health. More recently, scientists have also discovered that use of oral contraceptives may be linked with inflammatory bowel disease—in particular, an increased risk of Crohn's disease, which is characterized by inflammation of the lining and wall of the large or small intestine, or both.[16] The lining can become so inflamed that it bleeds.

Although the exact mechanism of this association is unknown, the current thinking is that the hormones change the permeability of the intestinal lining, as the colon has been shown to be more vulnerable to inflammation when hormones like estrogen are given. (This may also be why some women on birth control complain of gastrointestinal problems.) We know what increased permeability means for human health: it heightens the chance that materials from the intestine, especially those produced by gut bacteria, will end up in the bloodstream, where they incite the immune system, and can then move to other parts of the body, including the brain, where they inflict harm. In a 2012 study led by Dr. Hamed Khalili, a clinical and research fellow of gastroenterology at Massachusetts General Hospital in Boston, researchers looked at the data taken from about 233,000 women enrolled in the large U.S. Nurses Health Studies who were followed from 1976 through 2008.[17] Comparing those who never used birth control pills to those who did, he found that current users had a nearly three times greater risk of Crohn's disease. In his conclusions, Dr. Khalili warned that women on birth control pills who have a strong family history of inflammatory bowel disease should especially be made aware of the research finding a link between the two.

So what are the other options? Dr. Brogan, an advocate for women's health, wants all of her patients off oral contraceptives. She recommends that they try a non-hormonal intrauterine device (IUD), fertility gadgets that track a woman's body temperature accurately enough to know when ovulation is occurring, or the old-fashioned condom. In her words: "There's just no free lunch with medication treatment, and a risk/benefit analysis is very difficult to do if we don't know what environmental and genetic risks an individual is bringing to the table. If there is a treatment option that presents minimal to no appreciable risks and some degree of evidence-based benefit, this, to me, would represent the kinder, gentler road to health. These days, women's lib looks a lot more like a healthy, happy menstrual cycle free from the grips of a prescription."[18]

NSAIDS

In the past, multiple studies dating as far back as the 1990s have shown that people who have taken nonsteroidal anti-inflammatory medications such as Advil (ibuprofen) and Aleve (naproxen) for two or more years may have more than a 40 percent reduced risk for Alzheimer's and Parkinson's diseases.[19] This makes sense when you consider that these are principally inflammatory diseases, so when you control inflammation you control risk.

But newer studies are now emerging to reveal a twist in the story. It's been shown that these medications can increase the risk of damage to the gut lining, especially in the presence of gluten. Spanish researchers found that when mice that were genetically susceptible to gluten sensitivity were treated with indomethacin, a strong nonsteroidal anti-inflammatory that's often used to treat rheumatoid arthritis, there was a pronounced increase in intestinal permeability that amplified the damaging effects of gluten. Their conclusion indicated that "environmental factors that alter the intestinal barrier may predispose individuals to an increased susceptibility to gluten…"[20] Future research will help clarify this conundrum, but for now I'd caution against the use of these drugs unless they are truly necessary.

ENVIRONMENTAL CHEMICALS

Today there are an untold number of synthetic chemicals in our environment, many of them present in the things we touch, breathe, rub on our skin, and consume. Most individuals in industrialized nations now carry hundreds of synthetic chemicals in their body from air, water, and food. Traces of 232 synthetic chemicals have been found in the umbilical cord blood of infants at birth.[21] And the vast majority of these chemicals have not been adequately tested for health effects. In the last three decades, more than 100,000 chemicals have been approved for commercial use in the U.S., including more than 82,000 industrial chemicals, 1,000 pesticide active ingredients, 3,000 cosmetic ingredients, 9,000 food additives, and 3,000 pharmaceutical drugs.[22] The Environmental Protection Agency (EPA) and the Food and Drug Administration (FDA) only regulate a tiny fraction of these. In the years since the 1976 Toxic Substances Control Act (TSCA) was passed, funding constraints and industry litigation has meant the EPA has only been able to require safety testing on about 200 of the 84,000 chemicals listed on the TSCA chemical inventory. And of the 84,000, 8,000 are produced at annual volumes of 25,000 pounds or greater. So far, at least 800 of these chemicals are suspected of being capable of interfering with our hormonal system.

While we'd like to think scientists have been measuring industrial pollutants for decades and connecting that to human health, only recently have we begun to monitor the so-called "body burden," the levels of toxins in human blood, urine, umbilical cord blood, and breast milk. The vast majority of chemicals in current commercial use have not been fully analyzed for their effects on human health, so we don't know the true extent of risks from these chemicals or how they might disrupt the human body's normal physiology—and that of its microbiome. For this reason, it's prudent to be cautious and assume they are inflicting damage until we have solid research to prove otherwise.

One of the reasons environmental chemicals might be harmful is that they tend to be lipophilic, meaning that they accumulate in the endocrine glands and in fatty tissues. What's more, when the liver is overloaded with toxins to process, it can be less effective at clearing them from the body. This, in turn, changes the entire habitat of the body, as well as the microbial community.

A prominent concern among researchers lately is that a lot of chemicals mimic estrogen in the body, and we are exposed to many at once. For example, take the ubiquitous compound bisphenol-A (BPA). More than 93 percent of us carry traces of this chemical in our bodies.[23] BPA was first made in 1891 and was used as a synthetic estrogen drug for women and animals in the first half of the 20th century. It was prescribed to women to treat conditions related to menstruation, menopause, and nausea during pregnancy; farmers used it to promote growth in their cattle. But then its cancer-causing risks were revealed, and it was banned. In the late 1950s, BPA found another home when commercial manufacturers started putting it in plastics. This was after chemists at Bayer and General Electric discovered that when BPA was linked together in long chains (polymerized), it formed a hard plastic called polycarbonate, a material transparent enough to replace glass and strong enough to replace steel. Not long after that, it found its way into electronics, safety equipment, automobiles, and food containers. And since then, BPA has been used in many common products, from cash-register receipts to dental sealants. More than a million pounds of the substance are released into the environment each year. The BPA found in plastic food containers has been shown to generate hormonal imbalances in both women and men. Studies are now underway to see what kind of damage a chemical like BPA can inflict on microbial cells. While some studies have suggested that certain gut bacteria can degrade BPA, thereby making it less toxic to human cells, my concern is that BPA might favor the proliferation of those bacteria and result in a disrupted, imbalanced community.

BPA is just one of many chemicals we encounter in daily life. BPA may soon disappear from our commercial products and the food supply thanks to aggressive consumer lobbying, but thousands of other chemicals that can be equally as harmful will continue to flood our environment.

As I've said, it's impossible to know exactly how many synthetic chemicals we're exposed to today, and which ones are truly harmful to microbial and human cells. But it is better to err on the side of caution and try to lower your level of exposure to potentially noxious chemicals. This starts at home. In chapter 9, I'll cover all the steps you can take to minimize harmful exposures. The two in particular that should be avoided as much as possible are pesticides and chlorine. These have been shown to have detrimental effects on the gut bacteria. Pesticides, for one, are designed to kill bugs! And they are extremely toxic to mitochondria. Studies are now emerging that link popular pesticides with changes in the microbiome that in turn lead to health challenges from metabolic disorder to brain disease. One particularly disturbing study, published in 2011 by Korean researchers, discovered a disproportionate amount of methanogens, a type of microbe, in the intestines of obese women.[24] These researchers also measured what's called organochlorine pesticides in the women's blood, finding a remarkable pattern among the amount of pesticides in the blood, the level of obesity, and the volume of methanogens in the gut. The more "toxic" the person's blood, the more "toxic" the gut. Methanogens are notoriously linked not just to obesity, but also to periodontitis, colon cancer, and the intestinal disorder diverticulosis. The toxicity of pesticides is of such concern that below I'll further note why it's important to avoid most GMO foods due to their relationship with herbicides.

Chemicals found in our water supply, principally residual chlorine, can also be destructive to the microbiome. Chlorine is bactericidal; it effectively kills a large variety of microbial waterborne pathogens. Obviously, we don't want harmful or deadly microorganisms to be in our water. In fact, if there's one thing many of us take for granted today in the developed world, it's access to clean water. Chlorine is widely credited with ending outbreaks of waterborne disease in developed nations. Even *Life* magazine once called the filtration of drinking water and use of chlorine "probably the most significant public health advance of the millennium."[25]

However, municipal water tends to be overtreated, resulting in a chemical mixture that's toxic to the gut bacteria. Moreover, ingested chlorine can react with organic compounds to yield toxic byproducts that wreak further havoc. Based on studies of chlorine's effects on human cells, the EPA sets the safe level in drinking water at no more than four parts per million. Even that dilution can wipe out lots of organisms, as anyone knows who has killed a goldfish using tap water. In chapter 9, I'll offer ideas on how to avoid chlorinated water. It's easier than you think, and you won't have to call a plumber or invest in a water delivery service.

Even if we install air and water filters in our homes and minimize our use of all products known to contain suspicious chemicals, it's hard to control all pollutants. But we can, with relative ease, make a few shifts in what we purchase to limit our exposure to potentially harmful chemicals.

Another big concern regarding toxins in the environment is that we humans are at the top of the food chain. While that definitely has its pluses, it also means we're exposed to larger amounts of toxic substances through a process called bioaccumulation. Eating meat, dairy, and fish is one significant way in which we are exposed. For example, certain kinds of fish, such as swordfish, have a concentration of chemicals in their tissues exponentially greater than the concentration found in the surrounding water. On land, many livestock eat grains sprayed with pesticides and then store those toxic substances in their fat, along with potential toxins like hormones, antibiotics, and other chemicals. Consuming these products can expose you to chemicals used along the entire agricultural chain.

HERBICIDE-LADEN GMO FOODS

Let me preface this by saying that a lot of research still needs to be done on the potential health implications of genetically modified organisms, or GMOs. This is true whether we're talking about GMOs' direct biological effects on the body or their impact on the microbiome. By definition, GMOs are plants or animals that have been genetically engineered with DNA from other living things, including bacteria, viruses, plants, and animals. The genetic combinations that result cannot occur in nature or in traditional crossbreeding.

The top two GMO crops in the U.S. are corn and soy (and, by extension, all the products that contain these ingredients; it's estimated that GMOs are in as much as 80 percent of conventional processed food). In more than 60 countries around the world, including all of the countries in the European Union and Japan and Australia, significant restrictions or outright bans have been placed on the production and sale of GMOs. Here in the U.S., the government has approved them, and many people are rallying for better food labeling so they can choose to opt out of what some call "the experiment." One thorny matter: Many of the studies showing GMOs to be safe have been conducted by the same corporations that created and now profit from them.

As you can imagine, one of the major problems faced by farmers is the intrusion of weeds into their production fields. So rather than having to resort to manually removing weeds, an alternative has been created. America's farmers now spray a weed-killing chemical, glyphosate (RoundUp®), on their crops. The harvested crop is prevented from also being targeted by the herbicide because the seeds used are genetically modified to be resistant to the herbicide's effects. In the world of agriculture, these seeds are known as "RoundUp® ready."

The use of RoundUp®-ready GMO seeds has allowed farmers to use huge amounts of this herbicide. And it's happening globally. It is estimated that by 2017 farmers will apply an astounding 1.35 million metric tons of glyphosate to their crops.[26] But here's the problem: Glyphosate residues represent a threat to human health. In the wheat industry in particular, farmers saturate the fields with RoundUp® a few days before harvest to generate a bigger and better yield. This suggests a new perspective on the subject of gluten sensitivity: It just may be that the rise in gluten intolerance and celiac disease is largely due to the increased use of RoundUp®. When you chart the incidence of celiac and the levels of glyphosate applied to wheat over the past 25 years, a stunning parallel pattern emerges.[27]

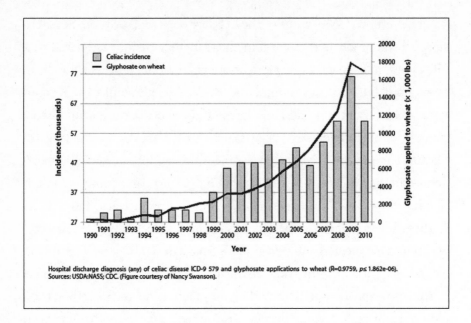

Hospital discharge diagnosis (any) of celiac disease ICD-9 579 and glyphosate applications to wheat (R=0.9759, p≤ 1.862e-06). Sources: USDA:NASS; CDC. (Figure courtesy of Nancy Swanson).

Mind you, correlation doesn't imply causation. While this chart seems to squarely show a relationship between the amount of glyphosate used on wheat (and presumably consumed through wheat products) and incidence of celiac disease, we cannot say that glyphosate *causes* celiac. That would be misinterpreting the data and making a false conclusion from just this evidence alone. But it's nonetheless interesting to note the parallel rise in celiac incidence and levels of glyphosate in the food supply. Many other variables are probably at play in this association, and for all we know there may be other factors going on in the environment to cause this surge in cases of celiac disease, but one thing we do know from recent research is that glyphosate does in fact impact the gut bacteria.

In a 2013 report published by the *Journal of Interdisciplinary Toxicology* from which this graph is taken, MIT research scientist Stephanie Seneff and an independent colleague came out with guns blazing about the effects of glyphosate in the body (they went so far as to argue that the practice of "ripening" sugar cane with glyphosate could be behind a recent surge in kidney failure among agricultural workers in Central America).[28] They pointed out that among glyphosate's effects on the body, it inhibits the cytochrome P450 (CYP) enzymes produced by the gut bacteria. These enzymes are critical to our biology, as they detoxify a multitude of foreign chemical compounds. If the CYP enzymes are missing, there's a much greater likelihood for that intestinal wall to become compromised and for harmful substances to find their way into the bloodstream.

In the report's plea for new policies regarding the safety of glyphosate residues in foods, it describes how residual glyphosate changes the composition of gut bacteria and wreaks havoc on human physiology. I'll spare you the biochemistry, but glyphosate

- compromises our ability to detoxify toxins

- impairs the function of vitamin D, an important hormonal key to brain health

- depletes iron, cobalt, molybdenum, and copper

- impairs the synthesis of tryptophan and tyrosine (important amino acids in protein and neurotransmitter production)

The scientists' report focuses on the link between glyphosate and celiac disease. They describe how fish that are exposed to glyphosate develop digestive problems that are comparable with celiac disease. And we know that celiac disease is associated with imbalances in gut bacteria. In fact, the scientists imply that glyphosate is the most important causal factor in the rise of gluten sensitivity through its known effects on gut bacteria. They conclude by stating, "We urge governments globally to reexamine their policy towards glyphosate and to introduce new legislation that would restrict its usage."

GMO CLAIMS: TRUE OR FALSE?

Currently, the FDA doesn't mandate GMO labeling, but many food manufacturers make non-GMO claims on their products. Can you trust the labeling? In 2014, Consumer Reports put these labels to the test, investigating more than 80 processed foods made with corn or soy and finding that the Non-GMO Project Verified seal, the Department of Agriculture organic seal, and other certified organic claims were, for the most part, reliable.[29] The most misleading claim, however, was "natural." Unless it had a non-GMO or certified-organic stamp of approval, "the food almost always had considerable levels of GMOs."

Don't panic. I'll help you clean up your environment and make gut-friendly choices—organic, grass-fed whenever possible, high-quality fats, and low-carb foods free of toxic ingredients. That's the whole point of my Brain Maker Rehab Program in part III.

PART III

BRAIN MAKER
REHAB

BRAVO. IF YOU'VE MADE IT this far, you've learned more about the body and brain and their intertwining physiology through the gut than most people in the world today, doctors included. You may have already thrown out your bread and thought about buying some oral probiotics. Or maybe you've dived headfirst into consuming yogurt daily and seeking foods marketed as containing "gut-friendly" strains of bacteria. No doubt you've picked up on some of the strategies I'm going to outline here in part III, which concludes with a 7-day menu plan.

Although my recommendations won't be terribly exacting, unlike what you'd find in a typical diet book with an explicit how-to in step-by-step fashion over the course of x-many days, my goal is to present ideas that allow you to tailor them to your tastes and preferences. I want to empower you to take control of your body and the future of your health. The suggestions offered here are more like general principles — guidelines for thinking through your lifestyle choices and personal circumstances in light of all this information. My recommendations should start you on your way to a vibrant, happy, healthy life, bright in mind and spirit.

Go at your own pace as you modify your diet and supplement regimen. Take as much time as you need to address your household environment and buy high-quality probiotics. But realize that the faster you execute these brain making recommendations and the closer you stick to them, the sooner you'll feel—and likely see—results. Indeed, this isn't just about transforming your health on the inside. Your complexion will glow. Your waistline will get smaller. And all those intangibles about you—your emotions, your energy levels, your ability to get things done and feel accomplished—will change for the better, too.

CHAPTER 8

Feeding Your Microbiome

*Six Essential Keys to Boosting Your
Brain by Boosting Your Gut*

I AM FREQUENTLY ASKED HOW long it takes to rehabilitate a dysfunctional or underperforming microbiome. Research shows that significant changes in the array of gut bacteria can take place in as little as six days after instituting a new dietary protocol, like the one I present in this chapter. But everyone is different; your Brain Maker rehab will depend on the current state of your gut and how quickly you can fully commit to making changes.

The following are the six essential keys to sustaining a healthy microbiome, based on the latest science.

KEY #1: CHOOSE FOODS RICH IN PROBIOTICS

For much of the world, fermented foods provide probiotic bacteria in the diet. Evidence suggests that food fermentation dates back over

7,000 years to wine making in Persia. The Chinese were fermenting cabbage 6,000 years ago.

Civilizations didn't understand the mechanism behind the fermentation process for centuries, but the health benefits associated with fermented foods were well recognized. Long before probiotics became available in capsules from health food stores, people have enjoyed one form of fermented food or another. Kimchi, a popular and traditional Korean side dish, is considered the national dish of Korea. It's usually made from cabbage or cucumber, but there are countless varieties. Sauerkraut, another form of fermented cabbage, remains popular throughout Central Europe. Then there are fermented milk products like yogurt that have been consumed for centuries around the world.

What is it that's so special about fermented foods? Fermentation is the metabolic process of converting carbohydrates like sugars into either alcohols and carbon dioxide or organic acids. It requires the presence of yeast, bacteria, or both. It occurs in conditions in which these organisms are deprived of oxygen. In fact, fermentation was described as "respiration without air" by the French chemist and microbiologist Louis Pasteur in the nineteenth century. Pasteur is renowned for his discoveries of the principles of microbial fermentation as well as pasteurization and vaccination.

While some of you may be familiar with the fermentation that takes place, for example, in the production of beer or wine, it's this same process that allows for the leavening of bread. Yeast converts sugar to carbon dioxide, and that leads to bread rising. (But we're not going to talk more about bread for obvious reasons. And no, it's not a probiotic.)

The type of fermentation that makes most foods probiotic (rich in beneficial bacteria) is called lactic acid fermentation. In this process, good bacteria convert the sugar molecules in the food into lactic acid. In doing so, the bacteria multiply and proliferate. This lactic acid in turn protects the fermented food from being invaded by pathogenic bacteria because it creates an environment with a low pH (i.e., an acidic environment), which kills off harmful bacteria with a higher pH. In the production of fermented foods today, for example, certain strains of good bacteria such as *Lactobacillus acidophilus* are introduced to the sugar-containing foods to jump-start the process. To make yogurt, for instance, all you need is a starter culture (strains of live active bacteria) and milk. Lactic acid fermentation is also used to preserve foods, extending their shelf life.

In the next chapter, I'll share details on what to look for in probiotic supplements, but there's no better way to consume a bevy of bifidobacteria and lactobacilli than to get them from wholly natural sources, which make them exceptionally bioavailable (easily accepted by the body). These are the strains that go to work in your body in numerous ways. They help maintain the integrity of the gut lining; balance the body's pH; serve as natural antibiotics, antivirals, and even antifungals; regulate immunity; and control inflammation. In addition, probiotic bacteria suppress the growth and even invasion of potentially pathogenic bacteria by producing antimicrobial substances called bacteriocins. What's more, as these probiotic bacteria metabolize their sources of fuel from your diet, they liberate various nutrients contained in the foods you eat, making them easier to be absorbed. For example, they increase the availability of vitamins A, C, and K, as well as vitamins from the B-complex group.

It was only at the turn of the twentieth century that Russian scientist Élie Mechnikov explored and revealed how *Lactobacillus* bacteria could be related to health. Mechnikov is considered the father of immunology, and one can argue that he's also the father of the probiotic movement. He won the Nobel Prize in Medicine in 1908. Remarkably prescient, he predicted many aspects of current immunobiology, and was the first to propose the theory that lactic acid bacteria are beneficial to human health. His ideas stemmed largely from recognizing a correlation between the longevity of Bulgarian peasants and their consumption of fermented milk products. He even went as far as to suggest that "oral administration of cultures of fermentative bacteria would implant the beneficial bacteria in the intestinal tract."[1, 2] And this was more than a century ago!

Mechnikov believed that aging was caused by toxic bacteria in the gut and that lactic acid could prolong life. He drank sour milk every day. He was a prolific writer, authoring three groundbreaking books: *Immunity in Infectious Diseases*, *The Nature of Man*, and *The Prolongation of Life: Optimistic Studies*, the last of which documented in detail the unusually lengthy life spans of several populations that regularly ate fermented foods and bacterial cultures called kefirs. He made numerous observational records of centenarians who were still leading active and healthy lives. And it was he who coined the term "probiotic" to describe beneficial bacteria. His work inspired twentieth-century Japanese microbiologist Minoru Shirota to investigate a causal relationship between bacteria and good intestinal health. Dr. Shirota's studies eventually led to the worldwide marketing of kefir and other fermented milk drinks, or probiotics.

The scientific community has finally caught up with Mechnikov's ideas.

In chapter 10, I'll share a wealth of recipes for creating delicious meals that use fermented foods. Let me list and describe the main ones here, some of which I've already mentioned.

- Live-cultured yogurt. An explosion of yogurt brands has taken over the dairy section lately, but you have to be careful about which brands to buy; many of them — both Greek and regular — are loaded with added sugar, artificial sweeteners, and artificial flavors. Read your labels. For people sensitive to dairy, coconut yogurt is an excellent dairy-free way to work plenty of enzymes and probiotics into your diet.

- Kefir. This fermented dairy product is very similar to yogurt. It is a unique combination of kefir "grains" (a combination of yeast and bacteria) and goat's milk that's high in lactobacilli and bifidobacteria. It's also rich in antioxidants. For those who are sensitive to dairy or lactose intolerant, coconut kefir, a non-dairy version, is also delicious and equally beneficial.

- Kombucha tea. This is a form of fermented black tea that has been used for centuries. Fizzy and often served chilled, it's also believed to help increase energy, and even help you lose weight.

- Tempeh. Many people, especially vegetarians, eat tempeh as a substitute for meat. Tempeh is fermented soybeans and is a complete protein, with all of the amino acids. Overall, I'm not a huge fan of soy products for a number of reasons, but small amounts of tempeh are acceptable. A great source of vitamin B12, tempeh can be crumbled over salads.

- Kimchi. In addition to providing beneficial bacteria, kimchi is also a great source of calcium, iron, beta-carotene, and vitamins A, C, B1, and B2. The only problem for some is that it's spicy. But it's one of the best probiotic foods you can add to your diet if you can handle the heat.

- Sauerkraut. Not only does this fermented cabbage fuel healthy gut bacteria, but it also contains choline, a chemical needed for the proper transmission of nerve impulses from the brain through the central nervous system.

- Pickles. No wonder many pregnant women crave pickles, one of the most basic and beloved natural probiotics. For many, pickles can be your gateway food to other, more exotic fermented foods.

- Pickled fruits and vegetables. Pickling fruits and veggies, such as carrot sticks, transforms the usual into the extraordinary. Whether you do this yourself or buy pickled produce, keep in mind that the probiotic benefits are only present in unpasteurized foods pickled in brine, not vinegar.

- Cultured condiments. Believe it or not, you can create lacto-fermented mayonnaise, mustard, horseradish, hot sauce, relish, salsa, guacamole, salad dressing, and fruit chutney. Sour cream, while technically a fermented dairy product, tends to lose its probiotic power during processing. Some manufacturers, however, add live cultures at the end of the process; look for these brands.

- Fermented meat, fish, and eggs. If you don't believe me, turn to page 244 for mouth-watering recipes from corned beef to pickled sardines and fermented hard-boiled eggs.

As a general note, if you're not going to make these dishes at home (using my easy recipes starting on page 225), be mindful of which products you buy in the market. Look out for added sugars, chemical preservatives, and colorings. Ideally, choose organic.

KEY #2: GO LOW-CARB, EMBRACE HIGH-QUALITY FAT

As *Homo sapiens*, we are virtually identical to every human that has walked on this planet. And we as a species have been shaped by nature over thousands of generations. For the greater part of the past 2.6 million years, our ancestors' diets consisted of wild animals and seasonal fruits and vegetables. Today most people's diets are centered on grains and carbs—many of which contain gut-blasting, microbiome-damaging gluten whose downstream effects reach the brain.

Even setting aside the gluten factor, one of the main reasons that consuming too many grains and carbs is so harmful is that they spike blood sugar in ways other foods, such as meat, fish, poultry, and vegetables, do not. I've already presented the facts on what excess blood sugar does to the body and the balance of gut bacteria. The more sugars consumed—even artificial ones—the sicker the microbiome becomes.

From a purely technological standpoint, we've come a long way since the Paleolithic era, but millions of us still suffer needlessly and struggle with our health. The fact that preventable, non-communicable diseases account for more deaths worldwide today than all other diseases combined is unacceptable. How can that be? We're living longer than previous generations, but not necessarily better. We've failed at averting and curing illnesses that we're susceptible to when we're older. I don't know anyone who wants to live to be 100 if their last twenty years are spent in misery.

It's clear to me that the shift in our diet over the past century is at fault for many of our modern scourges. As we went from eating a high-fat, high-fiber, low-carb diet to a low-fat, low-fiber, high-carb one, we concomitantly began to suffer from chronic conditions linked to the brain.

While it may be hard to believe, your brain, however smart and tech-savvy you are, isn't too dissimilar from the brain of an ancient ancestor born tens of thousands of years ago. Both evolved to seek out foods high in fat and sugar—a primal survival mechanism. Your caveman counterpart spent a long time hunting for food, and ate only meat (high in fat), fish, and the occasional natural sugar from plants and, if the season was right, fruits. Your hunting efforts end quickly because you have abundant access to processed fats and sugars. You and your caveman counterpart have brains that operate the same way, but your sources of nutrition are anything but the same.

You know by now that diets high in sugar and low in fiber fuel unwanted bacteria and increase the chances of intestinal permeability, mitochondrial damage, immune-system compromise, and widespread inflammation that reaches the brain. And it's a vicious cycle; all of these effects further assault that microbial balance.

A central premise in *Grain Brain* is the fact that fat—not carbohydrate—is the preferred fuel of human metabolism and has been for all of human evolution. I made my case for choosing high-quality fats and not worrying about so-called "high-cholesterol" foods. Let me summarize the main points here to put this into the context of the microbiome.

The famous Framingham Heart Study is one of the most treasured and revered studies ever performed in the United States. It has added reams of data to our understanding of certain risk factors for diseases. Although it was originally designed to identify common factors or characterstics that contribute to cardiovascular disease, it has since revealed risk factors for numerous conditions, including brain-related diseases. It has also brought to light the relationships between physical traits and genetic patterns.

Among the many illuminating studies that have come out of the original Framingham study was one conducted in the mid-2000s by researchers at Boston University, who analyzed the relationship between total cholesterol level and cognitive performance. They examined 789 men and 1,105 women, all of whom were free of dementia and stroke at the beginning of the study and were followed for sixteen to eighteen years. Every four to six years, cognitive tests were done to evaluate features that are compromised in people with Alzheimer's disease, features such as memory, learning, concept formation, concentration, attention, abstract reasoning, and organizational abilities.

According to the study's report, published in 2005, "lower naturally occurring total cholesterol levels are associated with poor performance on cognitive measures, which placed high demand on abstract reasoning, attention/concentration, word fluency, and executive functioning."[3] In other words, the people who had the *highest* cholesterol levels performed better on cognitive tests than those with lower levels. This pointed to a protective factor when it comes to cholesterol and the brain.

The newest research from around the world continues to flip old wisdom on its head. Coronary artery disease, a leading cause of heart attacks, may have more to do with inflammation than with high cholesterol. And the reasoning behind this has to do with cholesterol's role as a critical brain nutrient essential to the function of neurons. It also plays a fundamental part in building cellular membranes. Moreover, cholesterol acts as an antioxidant and a precursor to important brain-supporting molecules like vitamin D, as well as the steroid-related hormones (e.g., sex hormones such as testosterone and estrogen). The brain demands high amounts of cholesterol as a source of fuel, but neurons cannot themselves generate significant amounts of it. So they depend on cholesterol that's delivered by the bloodstream via a special carrier protein called LDL, or low-density lipoprotein. This is the same protein that's often demonized as being "bad cholesterol." But there's nothing bad about LDL, which is not a cholesterol molecule at all, good or bad. It's a vehicle for transporting life-sustaining cholesterol from the blood to the brain's neurons.

All of the latest science shows that when cholesterol levels are low, the brain simply doesn't function optimally. People with low cholesterol are at much greater risk for neurological problems from depression to dementia. One of the first studies to determine the difference in fat content between an Alzheimer's brain and a healthy brain was conducted by Danish researchers and published in 1998. In their study on deceased patients, scientists found that the people with Alzheimer's had significantly reduced amounts of fats in their cerebrospinal fluid, notably cholesterol and free fatty acids, than did the controls.[4] This was true regardless of whether the Alzheimer's patients had the defective gene — known as apoE4 — that predisposes people to the disease.

Given the established links that I've covered between excess weight, blood sugar control, and risk for brain disease, studies that examine the effects of various diets have also been revealing. One illuminating study in particular was published in the *Journal of the American Medical Association* in 2012.[5] In this study, Harvard researchers showed the effects of three popular diets on a group of overweight or obese young adults. The study's participants tried each of the diets for a month. One of the diets was low-fat (60 percent of the calories came from carbohydrates,

20 percent from fat, and 20 percent from protein); one was low-glycemic (40 percent of the calories came from carbohydrates, 40 percent from fat, and 20 percent from protein); and the third was very low in carbohydrates (10 percent of the calories came from carbohydrates, 60 percent from fat, and 30 percent from protein). Although all of the diets provided the same number of calories, the results were telling. Those on the low-carb, high-fat diet burned the most calories. The study also evaluated participants' insulin sensitivity during the four-week period while on each diet. They found that the low-carb diet triggered the most significant improvement in insulin sensitivity—almost twice that of the low-fat diet. The authors of the study also pointed out that people on the low-fat diet showed changes in blood chemistry that left them vulnerable to weight gain. They concluded that the best diet for maintaining weight loss is a low-carbohydrate, high-fat one. In other words, from the perspective of reducing risk for brain disease given the link between overweight/obesity and neurological disorders, the best diet is a low-carb, high-fat one.

If you haven't been able to connect the dots between low-carb, high-fat, high-fiber, and the microbiome, let me spell it out for you. This particular diet supplies the ingredients to nourish not only healthy biology (and thus a healthy microbiome) but also a healthy brain. A diet that keeps blood sugar balanced keeps gut bacteria balanced. A diet high in rich sources of fiber, which you'll get from whole fruits and vegetables, feeds the good gut bacteria and produces the right balance of those short-chain fatty acids to keep the gut lining in check. A diet devoid of injurious gluten will further tip the scales in favor of healthy gut ecology as well as healthy brain physiology. And a diet that's intrinsically anti-inflammatory is good for the gut and brain.

What exactly are the allowable ingredients on this diet? The menu plans and recipes in chapter 10 will help you follow this protocol, but let me give you a cheat sheet to guide you in shopping for and planning your meals. Note that the Brain Maker diet calls for the main entrée to be mostly fibrous fruits and vegetables that grow above ground, with protein as a side dish. Far too often people think a low-carb diet is all about eating copious amounts of meat and other sources of protein. On the contrary, an ideal plate in the Brain Maker protocol is a sizeable portion of vegetables (two-thirds of your plate) and about 3 to 4 ounces of protein. Meat and animal products should be a side dish, not a main course. You'll get your fats from those found naturally in protein, from ingredients used to prepare the protein dish and vegetables, such as butter and olive oil, and from nuts and seeds. The beauty of the Brain Maker diet is that you don't have to worry about portion control. If you focus on what you eat and stick to these guidelines, your body's natural appetite control systems kick into gear and you eat the right amount for your body and energy needs.

Brain Maker Foods:

- **Vegetables**: leafy greens and lettuces, collards, spinach, broccoli, kale, chard, cabbage, onions, mushrooms, cauliflower, Brussels sprouts, artichoke, alfalfa sprouts, green beans, celery, bok choy, radishes, watercress, turnip, asparagus, garlic, leek, fennel, shallots, scallions, ginger, jicama, parsley, water chestnuts

- **Low-sugar fruit**: avocado, bell peppers, cucumber, tomato, zucchini, squash, pumpkin, eggplant, lemons, limes

- **Fermented foods**: yogurt, pickled fruits and vegetables, kimchi, sauerkraut, fermented meat, fish, and eggs (see Key #1, page 179)

- **Healthy fat**: extra-virgin olive oil, sesame oil, coconut oil, grass-fed tallow and organic or pasture-fed butter, ghee, almond milk, avocados, coconuts, olives, nuts and nut butters, cheese (except for blue cheeses), and seeds (flaxseed, sunflower seeds, pumpkin seeds, sesame seeds, chia seeds)

- **Protein**: whole eggs; wild fish (salmon, black cod, mahimahi, grouper, herring, trout, sardines); shellfish and mollusks (shrimp, crab, lobster, mussels, clams, oysters); grass-fed meat, fowl, poultry, and pork (beef, lamb, liver, bison, chicken, turkey, duck, ostrich, veal); wild game

- **Herbs, seasonings, and condiments**: mustard, horseradish, tapenade, and salsa if they are free of gluten, wheat, soy, and sugar (kiss ketchup goodbye); no restrictions on herbs and seasonings (but be mindful of packaged products that may have been made at plants that process wheat and soy)

The following can be used in moderation ("moderation" means eating small amounts of these ingredients once a day or, ideally, just a couple times a week):

- Carrots and parsnips

- Cow's milk and cream: Use sparingly in recipes, coffee, and tea

- Legumes (beans, lentils, peas). Exception: chickpeas (hummus is fine)

- Non-gluten grains: amaranth, buckwheat, rice (brown, white, wild), millet, quinoa, sorghum, teff. Make sure any oats you buy are truly gluten-free; some come from plants that process wheat products, causing contamination. I generally recommend limiting non-gluten grains because when they are processed for human consumption (e.g., milling whole oats and preparing rice for packaging), their physical structure can change, and this may increase the risk of an inflammatory reaction

- Sweeteners: natural stevia and chocolate (see below about chocolate)

- Whole sweet fruit: Berries are best; be extra cautious of sugary fruits such as apricots, mangos, melons, papayas, plums (or prunes), and pineapples.

Remember to choose organic wherever possible and non-GMO, gluten-free foods (for a list of places where gluten hides, see my website). When you eat beef and poultry, choose antibiotic-free, grass-fed, 100-percent organic meats. Choose wild fish, which often have lower levels of toxins than farmed fish (for a list of sustainably caught fish that contain the lowest amounts of toxins, visit the Monterey Bay Aquarium's Seafood Watch at www.seafoodwatch.org). Remember to be cautious of products labeled "gluten-free" that are filled with processed ingredients and that are low in real nutrients. The goal is to choose foods that are naturally gluten-free, not products whose gluten has been processed out of the food.

KEY #3: ENJOY WINE, TEA, COFFEE, AND CHOCOLATE

You should rejoice in the fact you can embrace wine, coffee, and chocolate in moderation and tea to your heart's desire. They contain nature's best medicine for supporting the health of gut bacteria. Let me explain.

Flavonoids are produced by plants to protect themselves against such perpetrators as free radicals. They are polyphenols, powerful antioxidants found in plants; they may in fact be the most abundant antioxidant in the human diet. They are the subject of intensive research in the areas of cardiovascular disease, osteoporosis, cancers, and diabetes, as well as in the prevention of neurodegenerative conditions. In multiple studies, adding polyphenols to the diet has been shown to significantly reduce markers of oxidative stress, which in turn reduces the risk for neurological ailments. The main dietary sources of polyphenols are fruits and vegetables; plant-derived beverages, including coffee, red wine, and tea; and chocolate.

Polyphenols found in black tea are now being explored for their ability to positively influence gut microbial diversity.[6] Researchers are now able to quantify changes in gut bacteria when introducing a particular substance into the diet. The polyphenols in black tea have been shown to increase bifidobacteria, which help stabilize gut permeability; this may explain why black tea has anti-inflammatory properties.[7] Green tea has also been shown to increase bifidobacteria, while at the same time reducing levels of potentially harmful clostridial species.[8]

In one particularly prominent four-week study, subjects received either a high or low dose of flavonoids from the cocoa plant. Fecal samples were obtained before and after the interventions, and the types and array of bacteria were measured along with other physiologic markers. The group that consumed high doses of flavonoids had striking increases in bifidobacteria as well as lactobacilli species, along with pronounced decreases in Clostridia counts. These changes in gut bacteria were accompanied by an unmistakable reduction in C-reactive protein, that famous marker of inflammation associated with risk for disease.

In their paper, the authors note that these plant-derived compounds act like prebiotics—feeding the beneficial bacteria. They also point out that one of the species of Clostridia that was radically reduced was *Clostridium histolyticum*. This is among the species of Clostridia that are found to be increased in the stool of autistic patients. The authors indicated that the bacterial changes they observed were essentially the same as in studies done to examine the benefits of breast milk. Italian researchers, for another example, have demonstrated that in elderly individuals suffering from mild cognitive impairment, those who consumed the highest level of flavonoids from cocoa and chocolate improved their insulin sensitivity and blood pressure significantly. They also showed less free radical damage and heightened cognitive function.[9]

Other studies have not only confirmed these findings but have also shown that consuming flavonoids leads to significant improvement in blood flow to the brain.[10, 11] This is an important discovery, as a lot of new research now shows that people with dementia have less blood flow to the brain.

Like chocolate, coffee packs a healthy punch and has gained fame in the past couple of years thanks to new science highlighting its impact on the microbiome. I mentioned some of coffee's benefits earlier: it supports a healthy F/B ratio and exhibits anti-inflammatory and antioxidant properties. Coffee also stimulates a specific gene pathway called the Nrf2 pathway. When this is triggered, it causes the body to make higher levels of protective antioxidants, while reducing inflammation and enhancing detoxification. Other Nrf2 activators are chocolate (another bonus for cocoa), green tea, turmeric, and resveratrol, an ingredient in red wine.

Anyone who dines with me knows I love a glass. And in fact, drinking a glass of red wine a day can be good for you, and for your microbiome. Resveratrol, the natural polyphenol found in grapes, slows down the aging process, boosts blood flow to the brain, promotes heart health, and curbs fat cells by inhibiting their development. It also has a favorable effect on gut bacteria (they love their wine, too!). Spanish researchers have found that LPS levels, as a marker of both inflammation and intestinal permeability, were dramatically reduced in individuals who consumed red wine in moderation (one to two glasses per day).[12] Interestingly, the effect was the same even when the alcohol was removed. The researchers also analyzed the bacterial composition of the stool of such individuals and found a significant increase in bifidobacteria. Red wine is also a rich source of those gut-loving polyphenols. Just be sure that you don't drink too much. A glass a day for women, two for men at the most.

KEY #4: CHOOSE FOODS RICH IN PREBIOTICS

Prebiotics, the ingredients that gut bacteria love to eat to fuel their growth and activity, can easily be ingested through certain foods. It has been estimated that for every 100 grams of consumed carbohydrates that qualify as prebiotics, a full 30 grams of bacteria are produced. One of the benefits of having good bacteria in the gut is that they are able to use fiber-rich foods that we consume, which would otherwise be non-digestible, as a substrate for their own metabolism. As our gut bacteria metabolize these otherwise non-digestible foods, they produce those short-chain fatty acids we've discussed that help us stay healthy. As you'll recall, for example, butyric acid is produced, which improves the health of the intestinal lining. In addition, short-chain fatty acids help regulate sodium and water absorption and enhance our ability to absorb important minerals and calcium. They effectively lower the pH in the gut, which inhibits the growth of potential pathogens or damaging bacteria. And they enhance immune function.

Prebiotics, by definition, must have three characteristics. First and foremost, they must be non-digestible, meaning they pass through the stomach without being broken down by either gastric acids or enzymes. Second, they have to be able to be fermented or metabolized by the intestinal bacteria. And third, this activity has to confer health benefits. We've all heard about the benefits of eating fiber. It turns out that the effects of dietary fiber on the growth of healthy bacteria in the gut may well be fiber's most important aspect.

Foods high in prebiotics have been part of our diet since prehistoric times. It has been estimated that the typical hunter-gatherer in our distant past consumed as much as 135 g of inulin, a type of fiber, each day.[13] Prebiotics occur naturally in a variety of foods, including chicory, Jerusalem artichoke, garlic, onions, leeks, and jicama or Mexican yam; you'll see that I use these in many of my recipes.

Science has firmly documented many other health benefits of prebiotics:[14]

- They reduce febrile (fever-related) illnesses associated with diarrhea or respiratory events as well as the amount of antibiotics infants need.

- They reduce inflammation in inflammatory bowel diseases, and therefore help protect against colon cancer.

- They enhance the absorption of minerals in the body, including magnesium, possibly iron, and calcium (in one study, just 8 grams of prebiotics a day was shown to have a big effect on the uptake of calcium in the body that led to an increase in bone density).

- They lower some risk factors for cardiovascular disease, largely by reducing inflammation.

- They promote a sense of fullness or satiety, prevent obesity, and spur weight-loss. (Their effect on hormones is related to appetite; studies show that animals given prebiotics produce less ghrelin, the body's signal to the brain that it's time to eat. Studies have also shown that prebiotics like inulin dramatically change the F/B ratio for the better.)

- They reduce glycation, which increases free radicals, triggers inflammation, and lowers insulin resistance, and so compromises the integrity of the gut lining.

By and large, Americans don't get enough prebiotics. I recommend aiming for 12 grams daily, either from real foods, a supplement, or a combination thereof. Below is the list of top food sources of natural prebiotics.

- Acacia gum (or gum arabic)
- Raw chicory root

- Raw Jerusalem artichoke

- Raw dandelion greens

- Raw garlic

- Raw leek

- Raw onion

- Cooked onion

- Raw asparagus

While many of these may not appear easy to work with in the kitchen, my 7-day menu plan will show you how to make use of these ingredients and achieve the 12-gram-per-day minimum.

KEY #5: DRINK FILTERED WATER

To avoid the gut-busting chemicals like chlorine that are found in tap water, I recommend buying a household water filter. There are a variety of water treatment technologies available today, from simple filtration pitchers you fill manually to under-the-sink contraptions or units designed to filter the water coming into your home from its source. It's up to you to decide which one best suits your circumstances and budget. Make sure the filter you buy removes chlorine and other potential contaminants. Obviously, if you're a renter or live in a co-op building, you will be limited as to what you can do, but using filters on your faucets or pitchers with filters can work very well.

It's important that whichever filter you choose, you maintain it well and follow the manufacturer's directions to assure it continues to perform. As contaminants build up, a filter will become less effective, and it can then start to release chemicals back into your filtered water. You should also think about putting filters on your showerheads. Shower filtration systems are easy to find and inexpensive.

TIPS TO REDUCE CHEMICAL EXPOSURES

The dietary protocol outlined in this chapter will go a long way toward protecting you from a lot of unnecessary exposures to environmental chemicals, which can disrupt your microbiome and healthy brain physiology. Following are some additional ideas:

- Get to know your local farmers. Opt for locally sourced foods produced with the least amount of pesticides and herbicides. Check out the nearest farmers market and start shopping there.

- Minimize the use of canned, processed, and prepared foods. Cans are often lined with a BPA-laden coating, and processed foods are more likely to contain artificial ingredients like additives, preservatives, colorings, and chemical-based flavors. It's hard to know exactly what's in prepared foods you find at market buffets and in ready-made products. Cook from scratch so you know what's going into your food, but don't use nonstick pans or cookware. Teflon-coated wares contain perfluorooctanoic acid (PFOA), which the EPA has labeled a likely carcinogen.

- Don't microwave foods in plastic, which can release nasty chemicals that are absorbed by the food. Microwave in glass containers.

- Avoid storing food in plastic containers and plastic wrap made from PVC (which has the recycling code "3").

- Ditch plastic water bottles (or at least avoid plastics marked with a "PC" for polycarbonate, or the recycling label "7"). Buy reusable bottles made of food-grade stainless steel or glass.

- Ventilate your home well and install HEPA air filters if possible. Change your air conditioning and heating filters every three to six months. Get the ducts cleaned yearly. Avoid air deodorizers and plug-in room fresheners.

- Reduce toxic dust and residues on surfaces by using a vacuum cleaner with a HEPA filter. You may not see or smell these residues, but they can come from furniture, electronics, and textiles.

- Replace toxic household goods and products over time with alternatives free of synthetic chemicals. When it comes to toiletries, deodorants, soaps, and beauty products, finish using what you have and then switch brands. Look for the genuine USDA organic seal and choose products that are safer alternatives. A great resource for finding new brands is the Environmental Working Group's website at www.ewg.org.

- Keep as many plants in your home as possible that naturally detoxify the environment, such as spider plants, aloe vera, chrysanthemums, Gerber daisies, Boston ferns, English ivies, and philodendrons.

KEY #6: FAST EVERY SEASON

One critical mechanism of the human body is its ability to convert fat into vital fuel during times of starvation. We can break down fat into specialized molecules called ketones, and one in particular—beta-hydroxybutyrate (beta-HBA)—is a superior fuel for the brain. This provides a compelling case for the benefits of intermittent fasting, a topic I covered at length in *Grain Brain*.

Researchers have determined that beta-HBA, which is easily obtainable just by adding coconut oil to your diet, improves antioxidant function, increases the number of mitochondria, and stimulates the growth of new brain cells. And you know that anything that supports mitochondrial health and proliferation is good for brain health. These organelles, don't forget, are part of our microbiome.

Earlier I mentioned the Nrf2 gene pathway that, when activated, produces a dramatic increase in antioxidant protection and detoxification, as well as a decrease in inflammation. It also provides powerful stimulation for mitochondrial growth, and the pathway is turned on by fasting.

As you know, one of the most important processes in the body that is dictated by the mitochondria is programmed cell death, whereby cells commit suicide. It has only been in the last several years that researchers have finally delineated the steps in the cascade of chemical events that culminates in apoptotic cell death, which can be devastating if it's allowed to happen uncontrollably and leads to a loss of critical cells, such as those in the brain. Among the most widely recognized researchers in this area is Dr. Mark Mattson at the National Institute on Aging in Baltimore. Dr. Mattson has published extensively on the topic of reducing apoptosis to protect nerve cells. More specifically, his research has centered upon dietary habits, especially the role of calorie restriction in neuroprotection by its minimizing apoptosis, enhancing mitochondrial energy production, decreasing mitochondrial free radical formation, and enhancing mitochondrial growth. His work is compelling and gives us clear-cut scientific validation for the practice of fasting, a medical intervention described in the Vedic texts more than three thousand years ago. Indeed, we've known anecdotally for centuries that lowering caloric intake slows down aging, reduces age-related chronic disease, and prolongs life. But only recently has the science caught up with all the anecdotal evidence.[15, 16] In addition to the benefits I've already listed, calorie restriction has also been proven to increase insulin sensitivity, reduce the body's overall oxidative stress, trigger the expression of genes to manage stress and resist disease, and switch your body into fat-burning mode. All of these benefits in turn help sustain a healthy microbiome.

The idea of substantially reducing your daily calorie intake does not appeal to many people. But intermittent fasting—a complete restriction of food for twenty-four to seventy-two hours at regular intervals throughout the year—is more manageable and can achieve the same results as calorie restriction. Moreover, fasting can do something besides enhance the health and function of the mitochondria; it's finally being shown in laboratory studies that calorie restriction prompts changes to gut bacteria, which may also be responsible for some of calorie restriction's beneficial role in health. One prominent study, published in a specialty journal for *Nature* in 2013, demonstrated that calorie restriction enriches strains of bacteria that are associated with increased lifespan, and reduces those strains that are "negatively correlated with lifespan."[17] In their paper, the researchers noted that "animals under calorie restriction can establish a structurally balanced architecture of gut microbiota that may exert a health benefit to the host…" Even though these studies have looked at calorie restriction, remember that intermittent fasting provides comparable health benefits and is a more practical strategy for most people.

My fasting protocol is simple: No food but lots of water (avoid caffeine) for a twenty-four-hour period. If you take any medications, by all means continue to take them. (If you take diabetes medications, please consult your physician first.) When you've established this Brain Maker diet for life and want to fast for increased benefits, you can try a seventy-two-hour fast (assuming you've checked with your doctor if you have any medical conditions to consider). I recommend fasting at least four times a year; fasting during the seasonal changes (for example, the last week of September, December, March, and June) is an excellent practice to keep.

A NOTE FOR EXPECTANT MOTHERS

Pregnant and planning your birth experience? Speak with your doctor about using the so-called "gauze technique" if, for whatever reason, you undergo a C-section. Dr. Maria Gloria Dominguez-Bello has presented research suggesting that using gauze to collect a mother's birth-canal bacteria and then imparting them to babies born by C-section by rubbing the gauze over their mouths and noses does help make those babies' bacterial populations more closely resemble vaginally born babies. It's not a substitute for having a vaginal delivery, but it's better than a sterile C-section.

Plan ahead, too, for giving your baby the best nutrition possible. How effective are infant formulas that contain beneficial bacteria?

The benefits of human breast milk are so well established that formula companies strive to make their product resemble breast milk as much as possible—although the old adage still rings true: breast is best. What about supplementing traditional formula with probiotics designed for babies? The science in this area is still growing, but some studies have already shown that providing probiotics either through formula or as a supplement can have positive effects (I'll give specifics in chapter 9). They can reduce colic and irritability and lower the risk of infections that call for antibiotics. Certainly, they should not be considered a substitute for breast milk.

The intricacies of the microbiome are practically unfathomable. The microbiome is dynamic. It's ever-changing in response to our environment—the air we breathe, the people we touch, the drugs we take, the dirt and germs we encounter, the things we consume, and even the thoughts we have. Just as food gives our bodies information, so does our gut bacteria speak to our DNA, our biology, and, ultimately, our longevity.

While you may have come into the world naturally and breast-fed for at least six months, that doesn't mean you don't suffer from a sick microbiome today. Likewise, you may have entered this world through your mother's abdomen, been formula-fed, and yet enjoy vibrant health, thanks to the way you've been taking care of yourself—and your microbiome—over the years. It can cut both ways. Luckily, the suggestions in this chapter for ensuring the health of your gut bacteria work for everyone.

The beauty of the ideas in this chapter is that while the science may seem complex, adhering to these tenets is anything but. As soon as you open the door to the six essential habits that nourish and sustain a healthy microbiome, you will improve your entire body's chemistry—from the gut to the brain, and everything in between.

CHAPTER 9

Go Pro

The Guide to Supplements

WALK INTO ANY HEALTH FOOD store that has a supplement section and you're bound to be overwhelmed. And not just by the volume of options, but by the claims made on many labels. Indeed, this section can be tough to navigate. But I'm going to make it easy for you.

Before I get to the details of shopping for supplemental probiotics, let me share a story drawn from my own patient files.

Christopher came to see me when he was thirteen years old. He had been diagnosed with Tourette syndrome at age 6, when he began to experience tics—spontaneous, uncontrolled movements that are characteristic of this neurological disease of unknown origin. Although we don't know exactly how many people have Tourette syndrome, a CDC study has found that, in America, one out of every 360 children aged six through seventeen years has been diagnosed with Tourette syndrome. That translates to 138,000 American children overall today. Tourette syndrome affects all ethnic groups and races, but boys are affected three to five times more frequently than girls. Other issues commonly seen in Tourette patients include the following: ADHD in 63 percent, depression in 25 percent, autistic spectrum disorder in 35 percent, and anxiety in

49 percent. There's also a profoundly increased risk of Tourette syndrome in children with allergies. And allergies are a hallmark of an imbalance in the gut bacteria and an increased risk for a leaky gut. In fact, in one eye-opening 2011 study, a group of researchers in Taiwan performed a nationwide population-based case-control examination of people with Tourette syndrome. They confirmed that there is a damning correlation between this disorder and allergic diseases. For example, people with allergic rhinitis—signs of an allergy or hay fever as characterized by sneezing, watery eyes, itchy ears, nose, and throat—showed double the risk of Tourette syndrome. So unquestionably, the immune system is involved and something is going on there.

Back to Christopher. The clues quickly started to mount in my mind as I spoke with his mother. She indicated that his tics would occur when he consumed "certain foods, especially processed foods and foods that had dyes." At first, he made specific dietary changes that may, in fact, have been somewhat helpful, but still his situation worsened. And while he was born by full-term, vaginal delivery and was breast-fed for the first year of his life, he was treated with aggressive antibiotics for pneumonia at age three. Then, at age five he contracted a streptococcal throat infection that also required antibiotics. The following year he again had antibiotics for dental surgery.

Clearly, these events represented significant challenges to Christopher's gut microbiota. When I saw him, he was in the eighth grade and taking no medications. Although he'd been an excellent student according to his mother, his grades had recently started to decline. Christopher's examination was, for the most part, normal, with the exception of frequent obvious tics in the form of uncontrollable neck and head movements. His abdominal muscles would contract in a way that distorted his trunk, and I noted facial contortions as well. While people with Tourette syndrome often experience vocalizations—uncontrolled vocal sounds and repetitive utterances—Christopher didn't seem to have this problem.

Of all the clues to Christopher's condition, the one that turned the proverbial light on for me was his streptococcal infection years earlier. The medical literature is filled with studies that show a correlation between a previous strep infection and Tourette syndrome. Many of these children also have obsessive-compulsive disorder. In the literature, the phenomenon is called PANDAS, for Pediatric Autoimmune Neuropsychiatric Disorders Associated with Streptococcal Infections. The term is used to describe children who have these disorders and whose symptoms worsen following strep infections, such as strep throat and scarlet fever. I wasn't surprised to find that his blood work came back from the lab with elevated antibodies for strep. A normal level would be in the range of 80–150 units; Christopher's was 223. Much of the research in Tourette syndrome these days focuses on the role of this particular bacterium. (On a related note, antibodies to strep are also found to be higher in children with ADHD.) But as strep is a common bacterium that can infect us without long-term side effects once the immune system takes care of it, the question arises: What is it about the immune system in a Tourette patient that allows this bacterium to become an issue?

It seems that, for some people, there's a glitch in the body's immune response to this organism. One strong theory that researchers are pursuing is that the strep infection sets off an immune response which produces antibodies that do not attack just the strep. These antibodies also attack the brain, as they are unable to distinguish between the proteins found on the cell wall of the strep bacteria and those proteins found in the brain that are responsible for movement and behavior. Such a reaction puts Tourette syndrome in the autoimmune disorder category. It also puts it in the category of being a disorder rooted in inflammation. Studies that investigate this relationship have also called attention to the fact that cytokines—molecules that signal inflammation—enhance the activation of the stress response system in the body, which results in increased levels of cortisol. And cortisol increases gut permeability, which adversely stimulates the immune system and leads to more cytokine production that can impact the brain and trigger symptoms of Tourette syndrome. Moreover, researchers have documented a higher incidence of Tourette syndrome in those who have experienced psychosocial stress — circumstances that also result in increased cortisol production.

For Christopher, I knew that at the heart of his challenges was a dysfunctional gut. I discussed options for treatment with his mother. Mainstream medicine would choose to medicate him with potentially dangerous drugs, including antidepressants and antibiotics, depending on the individual symptoms and severity of the disorder. She didn't want to go down that road with her son, and she was certainly pleased that I was in her corner on that decision.

I soon found myself diving into a discussion about gut bacteria, explaining to both Christopher and his mother that it's very likely that Christopher's medical history had put a serious dent in the health and function of his microbiome. We spent a lot of time talking about his significant exposure to antibiotics and how that may have changed his immune system. And we had this discussion in the context of Tourette syndrome as an autoimmune disease, an idea supported by well-respected research.

Christopher and his mother were desperate. By now he was being ostracized in school and intimidated by his peers. His tearful mother was devastated by what was happening to her son, right on the cusp of his teenage years. I recommended to Christopher and his mother that instead of taking the probiotics orally, they consider using a simple drugstore enema enriched with six capsules of a probiotics supplement.

I have to admit that I was amazed that neither Christopher nor his mother seemed at all taken aback by my recommendation. As a matter of fact, they seemed to welcome it and were eager to get going. Following their appointment, they immediately went to a local pharmacy to buy the enema, and they proceeded to execute the plan. The next morning, my office received a phone call from Christopher's mother. The message was so important that my staff felt my appointment with another patient should be interrupted. I held my breath for a moment while getting to the phone. She told me that they did administer the enema and that within hours "his body had become more calm." She immediately asked me when they could do the next procedure and also if they could increase the dosage. I gave her the go-ahead, and she began administering 1200 billion units of the probiotics daily by enema. Christopher's Tourette symptoms virtually disappeared.

I present this story not to offer up a "cure" for the disorder, for every individual's case is different. Rather, I use it to illustrate the fundamental role of gut bacteria and the intricate connections between a mysterious brain disorder — in this case, Tourette syndrome — and the immune system. The fact that Christopher had elevated antibodies against a bacterium he was infected with long ago (and that his immune system should have successfully handled back then) was a clear indication that his immune system was flickering on abnormally and that this was also driving inflammation. These facts, coupled with Christopher's antibiotic history, made the choice in therapy a no-brainer, pardon the pun. Louis Pasteur famously said "Chance favors the prepared mind." I suspect Christopher's improvement and outstanding outcome could be deemed chance, but for someone like me, I'm glad I had the prepared mind to put him back on the path to health.

I often encounter people who say these ideas are really "outside the box," but I take this in a positive way. I explain that the real mission is not to keep thinking and acting outside the box, but rather to make the box bigger so that these ideas will become more widely accepted and serve to benefit many more people for whom our "standard of care" is failing.

PROBIOTICS: FIVE CORE SPECIES

The number of probiotics available today can be overwhelming. This industry didn't exist when I was going through medical school and during the early decades of my career. Now, the number of different combinations available at health food stores and even added to various foods is growing. There are thousands of different species of bacteria that make up the human microbiome. But some major players have been identified and aggressively studied in both animals and humans, and I'll focus on this core group.

To make the task of finding and purchasing the right formulas as easy as possible, I've simplified my recommendation to just five core probiotic species that are widely available: *Lactobacillus plantarum, Lactobacillus acidophilus, Lactobacillus brevis, Bifidobacterium lactis, and Bifidobacterium longum*. Different strains provide different benefits, but these are the ones that will, as we've been discussing since the beginning of the book, best support brain health in these ways:

- Fortifying the intestinal lining and reducing gut permeability

- Reducing LPS, the inflammatory molecule that can be dangerous if it reaches the bloodstream

- Increasing BDNF, the brain's growth hormone

- Sustaining an overall balance to crowd out any potentially rogue bacterial colonies

While there is some debate as to whether or not particular preparations allow the organisms to remain viable when taken orally, I'm confident that oral probiotics can effect meaningful change in the gut bacteria. That said, I must admit that in order to repopulate the gut with good bacteria and reestablish an effective barrier, I have had great success with variations of this core group of species administered directly into the colon using an enema. To be clear, this would be something you would need to discuss with your treating physician. But it's one of the most powerfully therapeutic interventions I have ever employed in more than 30 years of practicing medicine and in dealing with brain problems. (See page 211 for a step-by-step probiotic enema protocol.)

The probiotics industry is poised to explode. I am certain that, with time, other species of organisms will be identified that prove to be helpful and that they will make their way into various over-the-counter combinations. Don't be afraid to experiment with different combinations. But start by looking for the five particular species I've identified, because I do feel that these are the most important, given the scientific literature today. Keep in mind that if you are using probiotics, it's important to make sure you take in adequate prebiotics to allow these organisms to flourish and persist in the gut. You should get 12 grams a day by eating prebiotic foods twice daily. My meal plan will show you how to achieve this easily. Prebiotic fiber supplements are also available, and there are even pre- and probiotic combinations. It's critical to take probiotics with filtered water, otherwise you'll defeat their purpose. Chemicals, such as chlorine, that are added to many sources of water to kill bad bacteria will also kill good, probiotic bacteria.

To find the highest-quality probiotics, go to a store known for its natural supplement section and speak with the person most familiar with the store's array of brands (and who can offer an unbiased opinion). Probiotics are not regulated by the FDA, so you don't want to end up with a brand whose claims don't match the actual ingredients. Prices can vary wildly, too. The store rep can help you navigate all the nomenclature, as some of these specific strains are sold under multiple names. Most products contain several strains, and I encourage my patients to seek supplements that are marked *hypoallergenic* and contain at least the following species:

- *Lactobacillus plantarum:*[1,2] Found in kimchi, sauerkraut, and other cultured vegetables, this bug is one of the most beneficial bacteria in your body. It survives in the stomach for a long time and performs many functions that help regulate immunity and control inflammation in the gut. By virtue of its actions on pathogenic microbes, it helps prevent disease and maintains the right balance of gut bacteria to stave off the growth of rogue colonies. It also helps fortify the gut lining, fending off potential invaders that might compromise the intestinal wall and sneak into the bloodstream. In fact, *L. plantarum*'s beneficial impact on the gut lining is perhaps its most important attribute, for it reduces gut permeability, thereby reducing the associated risks for leaky gut—including an increased risk for virtually every brain disorder. Moreover, *L. plantarum* can quickly digest protein, and this has the ultimate effect of preventing food allergies and even treating such allergies when they arise. In animal studies, it's been shown to protect engineered mice from having clinical symptoms of multiple sclerosis, and it even reduced the inflammatory response typical of that condition. Finally, *L. plantarum* has an uncanny ability to absorb and maintain levels of important nutrients, such as brain-friendly omega-3 fatty acids, vitamins, and antioxidants. All of these actions make *L. plantarum* essential for fighting infection, controlling inflammation, and controlling pathogenic bacteria.

- *Lactobacillus acidophilus:*[3] *L. acidophilus* is the darling of fermented dairy products, including yogurt. It aids the immune system by keeping the balance of good vs. bad bacteria in check. In women, it helps to curb the growth of *Candida albicans*, a fungus that can cause yeast infections. *L. acidophilus* has also gained fame for its ability to help maintain cholesterol levels. In the small intestine, *L. acidophilus* produces many beneficial substances that combat pathogenic microbes, including acidolphilin, acidolin, bacteriocin, and lactocidin. It also manufactures lactase, which is needed to digest milk, and vitamin K, which promotes healthy coagulation of the blood.

- *Lactobacillus brevis:*[4] Sauerkraut and pickles owe a lot of their benefits to this bug, which improves immune function by increasing cellular immunity and even enhancing killer T cell activity. It's so effective in combating vaginosis, a common bacterial infection of the vagina, that it's added to pharmaceuticals used to treat it. *L. brevis* also acts to inhibit the effects of certain gut pathogens. And perhaps best of all, it has been shown to increase levels of that all-star brain-growth hormone BDNF.[5]

- *Bifidobacterium lactis* (also called *B. animalis*):[6] Fermented milk products like yogurt contain this gem, which is well documented to have a powerful effect on preventing digestive ills and boosting immunity. A study published in February 2009 in the *Journal of Digestive Diseases* found that healthy people who consumed a product containing this type of bacteria each day for two weeks reported improvements in digestive comfort compared to control subjects who followed their usual diet.[7] It's also known to be helpful in knocking out foodborne pathogens like salmonella, which causes diarrhea. What's really key about this bug is that it's been shown to boost immunity. In 2012, the *British Journal of Nutrition* reported a study in which people took a daily probiotic supplement containing *B. lactis*, another probiotic, or a placebo each day for six weeks.[8] They were given a flu shot after two weeks, and their antibody levels were measured after six weeks. Those who had taken either of the probiotic supplements had greater increases in antibodies than participants who took the placebo, showing that these probiotics may help improve immune function. Other studies have confirmed this finding.

- *Bifidobacterium longum*:[9] Just one of the 32 species that belong to the genus *bifidobacterium*, this is one of the first bugs to colonize our bodies at birth. It has been associated with improving lactose tolerance and preventing diarrhea, food allergies, and the proliferation of pathogens. It's also known to have antioxidant properties, as well as the ability to scavenge free radicals. In laboratory mice, *B. longum* has been shown to reduce anxiety. Like *L. acidophilus*, *B. longum* also helps maintain healthy cholesterol levels. In animal studies, *B. longum* has been shown to enhance BDNF production, just as *L. brevis* does. And some studies have shown that *B. longum* can help reduce the incidence of cancer by suppressing cancerous growths in the colon. The theory goes that since a high pH in the colon creates an environment that can promote cancerous growth, *B. longum* can help prevent colorectal cancer by effectively lowering the intestinal pH.

TRY A PROBIOTIC ENEMA, WITH PERMISSION

This won't be for everyone, but I can't tell you how many patients have benefited from this at-home procedure. It's the best way to introduce probiotic bacteria directly into the bowel. Enemas, one of the oldest remedies on the planet and dating back to the ancient Egyptians and Mayans, are used to flush out the lower bowel by injecting fluid into the rectum. (The word *enema* is Greek for "inject.") They are also used to administer certain medicinal therapies directly into the colon. It's imperative that you get clearance from your doctor before using an enema so that you don't harm yourself. Once you've gotten the go-ahead, here's what you'll need:

- Enema bag

- 3–6 probiotic capsules or 1/8 teaspoon powdered probiotic (Make sure they include bifidobacteria, as these are the dominant flora in the colon, whereas acidophilus prefer the small intestine.)

- Filtered (chlorine-free) water

- Lubricant (optional)

- Privacy

Plan to perform your enema in the morning after having a bowel movement. Fill a large cup with 12 ounces of lukewarm, filtered water. Break open the probiotic capsules and empty the probiotics into the water, stirring to dissolve. Fill the enema bag with the probiotic mixture, and close the bag using the clamp that comes with the device. Lie down flat on your side (either side is fine) on a towel or in the bathtub. Insert the nozzle tip into your rectum (use a lubricant if that helps). Holding the bag higher than the nozzle, release the clamp so the water flows into the colon. Try to hold the enema for 30 minutes if possible.

How often I recommend this procedure depends on the specific needs of the patient. In someone who has had aggressive antibiotic therapy, for example, I'd prescribe probiotic enemas as often as three times weekly for 4 to 6 weeks and then reassess the situation. Your personal treatment plan will depend on your own situation; ask your healthcare provider for a recommendation.

HELP, I'M TAKING ANTIBIOTICS

At some point, most of us will have to take a course of antibiotics to treat an infection. It's important to follow your doctor's prescription exactly (i.e., do not stop taking the drug even when you feel better, as this can spur new strains of bacteria that could potentially make the situation worse). Continue to take your probiotics, but do so "on the half time," meaning take them halfway between dosages of the antibiotics. For example, if you're instructed to take the antibiotics twice daily, then take the drug once in the morning and once at night, and take your probiotics at lunchtime. And be sure to get some *L. brevis* into the mix. Many strains of this bug are resistant to antibiotics, so *L. brevis* may be helpful in maintaining a healthy microbiome when taking prescribed antibiotics.

These days it seems like even minor bacterial infections are treated with powerful "broad-spectrum" antibiotics. I recommend having a discussion with your treating physician about identifying exactly which strain is causing the infection and using a more specific antibiotic to treat that particular pathogen.

WHAT CAN I GIVE A BABY?

Specially formulated probiotics for infants and toddlers are available. Ask your pediatrician which type he or she recommends based on your child's needs. These products typically come in liquid or powder form and can be added to breast milk or formula. Although more research is needed, we do have some evidence that probiotics for babies can help relieve common conditions such as colic, diarrhea, eczema, and general intestinal problems. A study published in *Pediatrics* in 2007, for example, found that colicky infants who took *Lactobacillus reuteri* saw results within one week.[10] By the fourth week, these babies were crying for only 51 minutes a day on average, compared with 145 minutes a day for the infants who were given simethicone, the active ingredient in many over-the-counter antigas products.

According to another study in *Pediatrics*, the probiotic group *Lactobacillus* (specifically, *Lactobacillus rhamnosus* GG, or LGG) has been shown to be effective in treating infectious diarrhea in children.[11] And in an ongoing Finnish study published in the *Lancet*, infants whose family members had a history of eczema or allergies were given either LGG or a placebo prenatally (that is, their mothers took the dose while pregnant) and until they were 6 months old. Researchers found that the children who took LGG were half as likely to develop eczema as those who took the placebo.[12]

Until a child is old enough to consume solid foods that contain probiotics, it helps to have these oral probiotics on hand. But make sure you discuss this with your child's pediatrician.

ADDITIONAL SUPPLEMENTS TO CONSIDER

In addition to the probiotics I recommend, I often encourage patients to add to their diet the following five supplements, all of which help sustain a healthy and balanced microbial community in the gut. Many of these substances, in fact, owe their benefits in the body to how they work in sync with gut bacteria.

DHA: Docosahexaenoic acid (DHA) is a star in the supplement kingdom and one of the most well-documented darlings in protecting the brain. DHA is an omega-3 fatty acid that makes up more than 90 percent of the omega-3 fats in the brain. Fifty percent of the weight of a neuron's membrane is composed of DHA, and it's a key component in heart tissue. The richest source of DHA in nature is human breast milk, which explains why breastfeeding is continually touted as important for neurologic health. DHA is also now added to formula as well as hundreds of food products. Take 1,000 mg daily. It's fine to buy DHA that comes in combination with EPA (eicosapentaenoic acid), and it doesn't matter whether it's derived from fish oil or algae.

Turmeric: A member of the ginger family, turmeric is the seasoning that gives curry powder its yellow color. It's long been known for its anti-inflammatory and antioxidant properties, and it's actively studied today for applications in neurology. New research shows that it can enhance the growth of new brain cells. In some people, it can even rival the antidepressant effects of Prozac. It's been used for thousands of years in Chinese and Indian medicine as a natural remedy for a variety of ailments. Curcumin, the most active constituent of turmeric, activates genes to produce a vast array of antioxidants that serve to protect our precious mitochondria. It also improves glucose metabolism, which is a good thing for maintaining a healthy balance of gut bacteria. If you're not eating a lot of curry dishes, I recommend a supplement of 500 mg twice daily.

Coconut oil: This superfuel for the brain also reduces inflammation, which is why it's known in the scientific literature to prevent and treat neurodegenerative disease states. Take a teaspoon or two of it straight, or use it when you prepare meals. Coconut oil is heat-stable, so if you are cooking at high temperatures, use this instead of canola oil.

Alpha-lipoic acid: This fatty acid is found inside every cell in the body, where it's needed to produce energy for the body's normal functions. It crosses the blood-brain barrier and acts as a powerful antioxidant in the brain. Scientists are now researching it as a potential treatment for strokes and other brain conditions that involve free-radical damage, such as dementia. Although the body can produce adequate supplies of this fatty acid, we often need to supplement this because of our modern lifestyle and inadequate diet. Aim for 300 mg daily.

Vitamin D: This is actually a hormone, not a vitamin. It is produced in the skin upon exposure to ultraviolet (UV) radiation from the sun. Although most people associate it with bone health and calcium levels, vitamin D has far-reaching effects on the body and especially on the brain. We know there are receptors for vitamin D throughout the entire central nervous system; we also know that vitamin D helps regulate enzymes in the brain and cerebrospinal fluid that are involved in manufacturing neurotransmitters and stimulating nerve growth. Both animal and human studies have indicated that vitamin D protects neurons from the damaging effects of free radicals and reduces inflammation. And here's a most important fact: vitamin D performs all of these tasks through its regulation of the gut bacteria.[13] Only in 2010 did we find out that gut bacteria interact with our vitamin D receptors, controlling them to either increase their activity or turn it down.

I encourage you to get your vitamin D levels tested and have your doctor help you find the optimal dose for you. Not everyone's will be the same. For adults, I generally recommend a starting dosage of 5,000 IU of vitamin D_3 daily. Some patients need more and others less. It's important to have your doctor track your vitamin D levels until you are able to identify a dosage that will keep you in the upper range of "normal" on the blood test.

One day, I trust we'll have more data to know precisely which probiotics and other supplements to take to treat x, y, and z. When I listened to Dr. R. Balfour Sartor, a distinguished professor of medicine, microbiology, and immunology and director of the University of North Carolina's Multidisciplinary Center for Inflammatory Bowel Disease, speak on the matter at a conference in 2014, he envisioned a time when synthetically created bacteria would be given to people with chronic inflammatory conditions. These probiotics would repopulate the gut in a targeted way, depending on the patient's specific disease. Imagine walking into your local health food store and finding remedies for obesity, ulcerative colitis, and depression sitting on the shelves. I can't wait for that day.

CHAPTER 10

The Brain Maker 7-Day Meal Plan

Eat Your Way to a Healthier Brain

IF THE THOUGHT OF EATING fermented foods and things like dandelion greens and kimchi sounds strange or somehow daunting, rest assured eating them will be an invigorating experience. And these foods are widely available today. I'll give you a week's worth of meal ideas to show you how plentiful your choices can be and how easy it is to incorporate natural probiotics from foods alone. You'll see an abundance of vegetables, fish, meat, poultry, nuts, and eggs. And you can easily craft simpler dishes based on the guidelines here (e.g., for lunch or dinner, pick a fish or meat to cook up with a side of raw fermented ["cultured"] vegetables and a green salad; for breakfast, pick hard-boiled eggs with a probiotic-rich yogurt). You'll also find a few ideas for appetizers, beverages, and condiments in the recipe section, which starts on page 225.

Every dish for which there is a recipe in this book is in boldface. Note: Many of the fermented dishes do require time to, well, ferment. So plan ahead! The fermentation process often needs certain basic ingredients, such as whey and brine, so it's good to have these already on hand

At www.DrPerlmutter.com/Resources you'll find my recommendations for specific brands of foods that follow my guidelines. Even though you'll be consuming more fermented foods daily and evicting gluten and most sugar from your diet, you'll be surprised by the abundance of options available to you. If there's any ingredient listed below that you don't recognize, my resources will contain guidance. Acacia powder, for example, may not be familiar to you now, but it can be found at most health food stores that sell supplements.

in large quantities. (Step-by-step instructions for making these basics are included here). I encourage you to read through all of the meal ideas and create a strategy to abide by the 7-day plan.

This plan is ultimately meant to showcase seven different days in the brain-making way of life; it's unrealistic to think you can follow this plan exactly to a T starting today and using homemade creations. Nonetheless, use the guidelines in the previous chapter and the ideas here to start building more brain-making meals right away. Until you finish making your own fermented foods at home, do your best to buy high-quality store-bought placeholders for now. And don't be afraid to make fair substitutions for foods you just don't like. If you don't care for salmon, for example, then substitute another wild-caught, cold-water fish, such as black cod. If kimchi is too spicy for you, choose another probiotic-rich side dish. I want you to have fun with these meals and enjoy the introduction to new flavors and cooking techniques. Remember, your aim will be to consume at least 12 grams of prebiotics. Dandelion greens, for example, are a rich source of prebiotics; buy a bunch of these greens for the week and add them to salads and vegetable dishes. To reap the benefits of acacia gum, you can buy acacia powder and mix it with water. Just 1 tablespoon will give you 6 grams of insoluble fiber—the kind of fiber the gut bugs love for their own nourishment.

When pan-frying foods, you can use butter, organic extra-virgin olive oil, or coconut oil. Avoid processed oils and cooking sprays, unless the spray is made from organic olive oil.

Also remember to choose grass-fed, organic, and wild whenever possible. I use only animal products from grass-fed animals because they are healthier for humans as well as better for the environment, the economy, and the farmer. For instance, grass-fed beef is low in saturated fat, but it also offers up to six times more omega-3 fatty acids. When choosing fish, don't forget: Aim to buy fish that has come in recently (ask your market's fishmonger), and use the Monterey Bay Aquarium's Seafood Watch website at www.seafoodwatch.org to further help you choose the highest-quality sustainable fish that contains the least amount of toxins such as mercury. All of the ingredients listed in the recipes were chosen because they are readily available in gluten-free versions, but always check labels to be sure. If you choose to buy a commercially made product, such as yogurt or sauerkraut, read the labels to make sure nothing but the finest ingredients are used (no extra sugar, additives, preservatives, etc.). Don't forget to visit your local farmers market to stock up on the week's freshest, organically farmed produce. Get to know your grocers; they can tell you what just came in and where your foods are coming from. Aim for choosing produce that's in season, and be willing to try new foods.

I've listed some snack ideas on page 223. When you're strapped for time and don't have access to a kitchen, which for many people is the case for lunch at work, pack food. Plan your meals in advance, and make larger batches to have leftovers.

Before you begin this 7-day plan, purchase your supplements—especially your probiotics. And consider doing one or both of the following: fast for the twenty-four hours before you begin, and try a probiotic enema on the morning of Day 1. That will get you started in a big way!

Each day, do your best to incorporate exercise into your routine. Aim to get your heart rate up for at least 30 minutes most days of the week. Go for a brisk thirty-minute walk in the evening or try a group exercise class. Your gut bugs will love it; they need the exercise, too. And they also need you to sleep well at night. Try to go to bed at the same time and get up at the same time every day over this next week (and beyond). You'll recall from chapter 3 that the gut bacteria have a big say in whether you can get a good night's sleep. As you rehabilitate your microbiome, see if the quality of your sleep improves.

THE 7-DAY MEAL PLAN

Day 1

- BREAKFAST: 1 cup **yogurt** (page 232) with crushed walnuts and blueberries; optional: coffee or black tea

- LUNCH: grilled king salmon with **preserved lemons** (page 252), with a side of leafy greens dressed in balsamic vinegar and olive oil; optional: **kombucha** (page 259) or green tea

- DINNER: 3 ounces steak topped with **pickled salsa** (page 257), with a side of greens and vegetables sautéed in butter and garlic; optional: glass of red wine

- DESSERT: 2 to 3 squares dark chocolate

Day 2

- BREAKFAST: 1 cup **yogurt** topped with **blueberry-mint preserves** (page 253); optional: coffee or black tea

- LUNCH: mixed-greens salad with 3 ounces grilled chicken and two **fermented hard-boiled eggs** (page 250), dressed in balsamic vinegar and olive oil; optional: **coconut water lemonade** (page 263) or **water kefir** (page 261)

- DINNER: 3 ounces steak topped with **pickled salsa**, with a side of greens and vegetables sautéed in butter and garlic; optional: glass of red wine

- DESSERT: half a cup of berries topped with a drizzle of unsweetened cream

Day 3

- BREAKFAST: 2 scrambled eggs with stir-fried onions, mushrooms, and spinach, and 1 cup **milk-based kefir** (page 230); optional: coffee or black tea

- LUNCH: stir-fried vegetables with **corned spiced pork loin** (page 245); optional: filtered water with 1 tablespoon of acacia powder (see resources) or **kombucha** (page 259)

- DINNER: 3 ounces **raw fish ferment** (page 249), with a side of greens and vegetables sautéed in butter and garlic; optional: glass of red wine

- DESSERT: ½ cup **quark** (page 233) with a drizzle of honey

Day 4

- BREAKFAST: 1 cup **yogurt** with fresh fruit and a sprinkle of ground flax seeds, with half an avocado drizzled with olive oil; optional: coffee or black tea

- LUNCH: grilled steak with **sweet cippolini onions** (page 240), with a side of roasted vegetables; optional: **kombucha** or **water kefir**

- DINNER: 3 ounces wild, cold-water fish of choice, with a side of **kimchi** (page 241) and steamed asparagus; optional: glass of red wine

- DESSERT: 1 whole piece of fruit with an optional sprinkle of stevia and cinnamon

Day 5

- BREAKFAST: 3 to 4 slices of lox or smoked salmon with **ricotta** (page 234) and 1 soft-boiled egg; optional: coffee or black tea

- LUNCH: Mixed greens salad with raw dandelion greens, diced chicken, and **spiced asparagus** (page 238), dressed with balsamic vinegar and olive oil; optional: **kombucha**, green tea, or **coconut water lemonade**

- DINNER: grilled or roasted meat of your choice, with a side of greens and vegetables sautéed in butter and garlic; optional: glass of red wine

- DESSERT: 2 squares dark chocolate dipped in 1 tablespoon almond butter

Day 6

- BREAKFAST: 2 eggs any style, with unlimited stir-fried veggies (e.g., onions, mushrooms, spinach, broccoli) and 1 cup **milk-based kefir**; optional: coffee or black tea

- LUNCH: roasted chicken with **pickled garlic** (page 256), with a side of leafy greens with dandelion, and ½ cup wild rice; optional: filtered water with 1 tablespoon acacia powder mixed in or green tea

- DINNER: **corned beef** (page 244) and **basic sauerkraut** (page 236), with a side of steamed vegetables drizzled with olive oil; optional: glass of red wine

- DESSERT: 1 piece of whole fruit of your choice dipped in 1 tablespoon melted dark chocolate

Day 7

- BREAKFAST: 1 cup **yogurt** topped with mixed fresh berries, shaved coconut, and chopped walnuts, with 1 traditional hard-boiled egg; optional: coffee or black tea

- LUNCH: mixed greens salad with shaved Jerusalem artichoke and 4 ounces of ahi tuna, dressed in balsamic vinegar and olive oil; optional: **water kefir** or green tea

- DINNER: **Scandinavian-style fermented salmon** (page 248) over mixed greens, with a side of vegetables sautéed in butter and garlic and ½ cup brown rice; optional: glass of red wine

- DESSERT: skip

SNACK IDEAS

- **Jicama pickle**

- Hummus with **pickled garlic** and celery sticks

- Shrimp dipped in **pickled salsa**

- **Fermented hard-boiled eggs**

- **Pickled sardines**

- Chopped raw vegetables (asparagus, leeks, bell peppers, broccoli, green beans) dipped in guacamole, goat cheese, tapenade, or nut butter

- Sliced smoked salmon or lox with a spread of ricotta

- Half an avocado drizzled with olive oil, salt, and pepper

- Nuts and olives

Following the Brain Maker dietary principles is easier than you think, and you'll soon get used to a lot of new and terrific flavors. Even though this lifestyle limits your intake of carbohydrates, especially wheat and sugar, there's really no shortage of foods and ingredients to play with in the kitchen. You'll have to get a little creative in preparing some of your beloved dishes that rely heavily on flour, wheat, and sugar, but over time you'll learn how to make substitutions, and you should soon be able to return to your classic cookbooks. I like to use coconut flour, nut meals (e.g., ground almonds), and flaxseed instead of regular flour or wheat. To sweeten a dish, try stevia rather than sugar. And cook with butter and extra-virgin olive oil, ditching the processed vegetable oils. After you've completed the 7-Day Meal Plan, make it a goal to incorporate at least one fermented food into your daily menu going forward. Repeat the 7-day plan when you feel you've strayed too far from the guidelines and want to reboot your microbiome again. Perhaps that might happen over the holidays, after a family wedding, during an acutely stressful period, or in connection with some event in your life that had you reverting back to old dietary habits. This protocol can be your lifeline to a healthier way of living at any given time.

The Recipes

BASICS

Whey

Makes 1 quart

Whey, the liquid left after milk has curdled and been strained, is often used as a starter culture in fermented recipes. Nonrefrigerated raw milk that has been left to sour will naturally form lumps and liquid known as curds and whey, as in the Miss Muffet nursery rhyme. As the curds drain, nutrient-rich whey remains.

When drained, organic whole-milk yogurt will exude liquid whey, leaving a thick cream-cheese–like substance that can be used as a spread. Whey is also produced when one makes homemade ricotta (see page 234) or other creamy cheeses, and this whey, too, can be used in fermenting. Whey assists in the production of the microorganisms that make fermented foods so good for you; it also decreases the amount of salt required for fermentation.

You can use either homemade or store-bought yogurt, as long as it has been produced with organic, full-fat milk (goat, sheep, or cow) from grass-fed animals and contains live cultures; however, do not use Greek yogurt, as much of the whey has already been drained off. You will need a large colander or fine-mesh sieve and unbleached cotton cheesecloth to prepare the recipe.

8 cups homemade or store-bought plain, full-fat yogurt from grass-fed cows, sheep, or goats (see page 232), brought to room temperature

Dampen enough cheesecloth to cover the interior of a large colander or fine-mesh sieve. Fit the cheesecloth into the colander, taking care that it completely covers it. Set the lined colander into a large glass bowl or nonreactive container large enough to allow a few inches of space between the bottom of the colander and the bottom of the bowl.

Spoon the yogurt into the colander, and set it aside at room temperature to drip for 4 hours or until a substantial amount of whey has drained into the bowl. Pour the whey into a clean glass container, cover tightly, and set aside. (It doesn't need to be refrigerated.)

Pull the cheesecloth up and around the firm cream that remains, and tie the ends together to make a tight bundle, creating pressure to continue the draining. Leave the bundle in the colander for at least another 8 hours or overnight or until no more liquid is draining off.

Combine the remaining whey with the jarred whey, cover tightly, and refrigerate for up to 2 months. Whey may be frozen for up to 3 months, but after that the microorganisms begin to die.

Place the cream-cheese–like remaining yogurt into a clean container, cover, and refrigerate for use as a cheese or spread. This may be stored, covered and refrigerated, for up to 1 week.

Kefir Whey

Makes 1 cup

Kefir is a fermented dairy product that is similar to yogurt but substantially thinner in consistency. The most noticeable difference between the two is that kefir starter consists of granular "grains" that are combinations of bacteria and yeast living in dairy components, and the microbes do best at room temperature. In contrast, yogurt is the result of the bacterial fermentation of milk, and its microbes thrive above about 100°F. Also, kefir is most frequently consumed as a beverage rather than eaten, as yogurt is.

> 2 cups plain homemade or store-bought organic milk-based kefir (see page 230)

Dampen enough cheesecloth to cover the interior of a fine-mesh sieve with two layers. Fit the cheesecloth into the sieve, taking care that it completely covers it. Set the lined sieve in a large glass bowl or nonreactive container large enough to allow a few inches of space to remain between the bottom of the sieve and the bottom of the bowl.

Pour the kefir into the sieve. Cover with plastic film, and place the bowl in the refrigerator. Let it drip for 8 hours or overnight or until all of the whey has dripped off and the kefir has thickened.

Transfer the whey to a clean glass container, cover, and refrigerate for up to 1 month, although the bacteria in the whey are most vigorous when freshly prepared. Scrape the thickened, cream-cheese–like kefir remaining in the cheesecloth into a clean container, cover, and refrigerate for up to 1 month to use as a cheese or spread. (Avoid freezing.)

Basic Brine

Makes 1 quart

Since many fermented foods require brine, it is a good idea to keep some on hand. The following recipe makes a minimal amount, but it may be increased incrementally to meet your needs. Refrigerated, brine will keep indefinitely.

Because the water is so important in fermenting, it is imperative that you use distilled water when making a brine. Most tap water has been treated with chlorine or chloramine, which kill the good microorganisms you need; well water may have chemicals or salts that will adversely affect the fermentation process; filtered water may still contain trace chemicals; and bottled water that is not labeled "distilled" may contain unwanted chemicals, too.

I recommend using only pure sea salt in brines and all forms of fermenting. Table salt contains undesirable iodine and chemicals, so it should never be used in brine, as it will impede fermentation and may lead to spoilage.

> 4 cups cold distilled water
>
> 3 tablespoons fine pure sea salt (or 4½ tablespoons coarse pure sea salt)

Combine the water and salt in any container with a tight-fitting lid, stirring to blend (the salt will eventually dissolve). Cover and refrigerate until ready to use. If the brine is needed immediately, dissolve the salt in 1 cup of very warm distilled water and then combine it with the remaining 3 cups of cold water.

Spiced Brine

Makes 1 quart

Spiced brine is used most generally for curing meats and fish, as the spices and sweetness add the complexity these recipes require. You may use any combination of organic spices and dried herbs that appeal to you so that you can make your own personal mark on a dish. All of the same information given for Basic Brine (see page 227) applies to making Spiced Brine.

4 cups cold distilled water

3 tablespoons fine pure sea salt (or 4½ tablespoons coarse pure sea salt)

2 tablespoons raw honey

2 organic bay leaves

¼ teaspoon organic black peppercorns

¼ teaspoon organic allspice berries

¼ teaspoon organic juniper berries

¼ teaspoon organic whole coriander

¼ teaspoon organic mustard seeds

Whole organic dried hot chiles or red pepper flakes to taste, optional

Combine the water and salt in a large saucepan with the raw honey, bay leaves, peppercorns, allspice, juniper, coriander, and mustard seeds. If heat is desired, add dried chiles or red pepper flakes to taste. Place over medium heat, and bring to a simmer. Remove from the heat and let stand until cool.

DAIRY

Milk-Based Kefir

Makes 1 quart

Kefir is an ancient fermented milk drink that originated in the Caucasus region between Europe and Asia and was made from camel's milk. Although it is now most commonly made from cow's milk, it can also be made from goat's or sheep's milk as well as unsweetened coconut or almond milk. With moderate fermentation, it is slightly sour and reminiscent of a faintly bubbly, liquid yogurt. It has been touted as the secret to longevity and superb health.

¼ cup kefir grains (see note below)

4 cups organic full-fat milk from grass-fed cows

Place the kefir grains in a clean, sterilized container, such as a 1-quart glass canning jar with a sterilized lid. Add the milk, tightly seal the jar, and set it aside at room temperature for 24 hours. After the initial fermentation, you can let it stand at room temperature for weeks, but remember that it will get increasingly sour as it sits and eventually become too sour to drink. Refrigerated milk kefir will last for months.

After 24 hours of fermentation, open the jar, and pour the liquid through a fine-mesh strainer into a clean container, reserving the kefir grains as directed in the note below. Return the kefir to the quart container, tightly seal, and place in the refrigerator.

The kefir may be consumed at this point or kept, refrigerated, for up to 1 year. However, the longer it is refrigerated, the more sour it will become.

At this point, if you wish to flavor the kefir, you can put it through a second fermentation period using the same container. Add whatever flavors you wish, such as fresh berries, cinnamon sticks, whole nutmeg, cardamom seeds, chai tea, or orange peel. It is difficult to give exact amounts of these ingredients, as that will depend on the strength of flavor you desire. The more flavoring you add, the stronger the flavor will of course be. But it is best to start on the low end; for example, ¼ cup of fresh berries, 1 to 2 pieces of a spice, 1 teaspoon chai tea, or the zest of 1 orange.

Combine the kefir with the flavoring, tightly seal, and set aside to ferment at room temperature for 12 to 24 hours; the longer you leave it, the more flavor it will absorb. The kefir may be consumed at this point or kept, refrigerated, for up to 1 year. Again, the longer it is refrigerated, the more sour it will become.

NOTE: Kefir grains are a yeast/bacteria mixture held together in milk proteins and complex sugars. They range in size from that of a small grain of rice to that of a hazelnut and incorporate friendly organisms into milk as it ferments. Since they are alive, they require continual nourishment. This means that after use, they should be stored in fresh full-fat milk, covered, and refrigerated. In a ratio of 1 tablespoon of grains to 1 cup of milk, they will remain active for a week. If you need to store them for longer periods, add 1 cup of milk (per tablespoon of grains) each week it is stored. Although it would seem that storing them this way would turn the milk into kefir, this does not happen because the cold inhibits the fermentation process. Kefir grains will also quickly die if they are exposed to high levels of heat, such as in a very hot freshly sterilized container.

When making kefir from coconut or almond milk, it will be necessary to refresh the grains in full-fat milk, as these alternative milks do not contain the lactose necessary to nourish them.

Yogurt

Makes 1 quart

Yogurt is very quick and easy to prepare. All you need is milk, yogurt starter, and some time. One of nature's original prepared foods, yogurt was probably discovered by the nomadic tribes of Asia and Eastern Europe when the milk carried in their sheep- or goat-skin pouches inadvertently fermented with the sun's warmth. Like kefir, yogurt is believed to be a factor in the extraordinary longevity of the people of the Caucasus region and Bulgaria.

To make yogurt successfully in the home kitchen, you will need an instant-read food thermometer and a yogurt maker, or a place that remains at a near-constant 110–115°F, such as a pilot-light–driven oven with a constant temperature of 110°F. Once you have made your own yogurt, always remember to keep ¼ cup from each batch to make the next one.

> 4 cups organic full-fat milk from grass-fed cows, sheep, or goats
>
> ¼ cup organic full-fat yogurt made from milk from grass-fed cows, sheep, or goats (see note)

Place the milk in a medium-size heavy-bottomed saucepan over medium heat. Bring to 185°F on an instant-read food thermometer, watching carefully to keep the milk from boiling over. Once the temperature has been reached, remove from the heat and set aside. Allow the milk to cool to 110°F. If you are in a rush, place the saucepan in an ice bath and stir to speed cooling, but do not allow the milk to get cooler than the required 110°F.

Whisk the yogurt into the warm milk until it is completely blended. Pour the mixture into clean, sterilized containers with sterilized lids, such as four 8-ounce glass jelly canning jars or a 1-quart glass canning jar; or, if using a yogurt maker, pour the mixture into its containers.

If using the jars, tightly cover, and place in a spot that remains at a near-constant 110°–115°F for 8 to 12 hours or until it reaches the tanginess and thickness that you desire. Transfer to the refrigerator and store for up to 2 weeks. If using a yogurt maker, follow the manufacturer's directions for that specific machine.

NOTE: Both sheep's milk and goat's milk tend to produce yogurts that are somewhat looser in texture than yogurt made from cow's milk.

Quark

Makes 1 cup

Quark, the German word for "curd," is a fresh cheese common throughout Europe. The texture achieved depends on the type of milk used and the length of fermentation. It can be as loose as sour cream or as thick as cream cheese. It can be flavored with herbs, aromatics, or citrus zest. Quite tangy, quark is used in sauces, dips, salads, and desserts. Like ricotta, it can be served as a dessert with a drizzle of honey, a piece of fruit, or a bowl of berries.

Once you have made your own quark, retain about ¼ cup from each batch to use as the culture in place of the buttermilk for your next batch.

4 cups organic full-fat milk from grass-fed cows, goats, or sheep

3 tablespoons organic full-fat buttermilk from grass-fed cows, goats, or sheep

Place the milk in a medium-size heavy-bottomed saucepan with a tight-fitting lid over medium heat. Bring to 165°F on an instant-read food thermometer, watching carefully to keep the milk from boiling over. Once the temperature has been reached, remove from the heat and cover tightly. Set aside for about 1 hour or until the milk has come to room temperature (no cooler than 70°F).

Uncover and whisk in the buttermilk. Again, cover and set aside for 18 hours or until the milk has clabbered (soured and curdled) and thickened into a slightly sour yogurt-like substance.

Dampen enough cheesecloth to cover the interior of a fine-mesh sieve with two layers. Fit the cheesecloth into the sieve, taking care that it completely covers it. Set the lined sieve into a large glass bowl or nonreactive container large enough to allow a few inches of space to remain between the bottom of the sieve and the bottom of the bowl.

Using a metal spoon, transfer the clabbered milk to the cheesecloth-lined strainer, cover with plastic film, and refrigerate for 8 hours or until the desired consistency is reached. You may have to stir the clabbered milk from time to time to keep the whey (liquid) flowing. Do not discard the whey; it may be used as a beverage or in any recipe requiring whey. Store the whey as directed on page 226.

Store the quark, covered and refrigerated, for up to 1 month.

Ricotta

Makes about 1½ cups

This recipe — which is so easy to make and so much creamier than most commercially made ricottas — will become a standard in your kitchen. It is useful as a spread, a component of salads, and a dessert with a bowl of berries or drizzled with a bit of honey or Blueberry-Mint Preserves (see page 253). Traditionally, northern Italians don't like their ricotta salted, while southern Italians prefer it salted. If you are going to use the ricotta solely as a dessert, you can flavor it with a tablespoon or two of honey when boiling the milk.

2 cups organic full-fat milk from grass-fed cows

1 cup organic heavy cream from grass-fed cows

½ teaspoon fine pure sea salt (optional)

1½ tablespoons strained fresh lemon juice

Dampen enough cheesecloth to cover the interior of a fine-mesh sieve with two layers. Fit the cheesecloth into the sieve, taking care that it completely covers it. Set the lined sieve into a large glass bowl or nonreactive container large enough to allow a few inches of space to remain between the bottom of the sieve and the bottom of the bowl. Set aside.

Combine the milk and cream and, if desired, salt in a heavy-bottomed pot over medium heat. Bring to a gentle boil and boil for 1 minute. Remove from the heat and stir in the lemon juice.

Set aside to rest for about 4 minutes or just until the mixture separates into visible curds and whey. Using a slotted spoon, transfer the curds to the cheesecloth-lined sieve, cover with plastic film, and set aside to drain for about 2 hours or until the desired consistency is reached. The longer you allow the mixture to drain, the denser the finished cheese. Do not discard the whey; it may be used as a beverage or in any recipe requiring whey. Store the whey as directed on page 226.

Scrape the ricotta from the cheesecloth, and place in a nonreactive container. Store, covered and refrigerated, for up to 5 days.

VEGETABLES

Basic Sauerkraut

Makes 1 quart

This is, perhaps, the easiest recipe to introduce fermenting into your life; nothing is needed but organic cabbage, sea salt, and time. You can use any type of cabbage—red, napa, savoy, Brussels sprouts—it really is up to you. Not only is it easy to make, but fresh sauerkraut is very good for you. It contains *Lactobacilli,* beneficial bacteria that aid in the functioning of the digestive tract, and it is an excellent source of essential nutrients and fiber. Refrigerated, sauerkraut keeps for a very long time, usually up to a year, without losing flavor. Fresh sauerkraut is best eaten raw, while mature, intensely flavored kraut is often best cooked.

To make sure that the ratio of cabbage to salt is correct, I recommend that you weigh the cabbage after you have removed the core and any wilted or damaged outer leaves.

2½ pounds organic cabbage, cored and with wilted or damaged outer leaves removed

3 teaspoons fine pure sea salt

Shred the cabbage into coarse threads using either a food processor fitted with the shredding blade, the large holes of a hand-held box grater, a mandoline, or a large, sharp chef's knife.

Place the cabbage in a large bowl, and sprinkle the salt over the top. Using your hands, begin massaging the salt into the cabbage, working until you have begun to easily squeeze liquid from the cabbage. The time required will depend on the freshness of the cabbage and the strength of your massage and can range from a couple of minutes to 30 minutes or so.

Pack the cabbage and the liquid into a clean, sterilized container, such as a 1-quart glass canning jar with a sterilized lid or a 1-quart crock with a sterilized, tight-fitting lid. Using your fingertips, a smaller jar or glass that will fit down into the larger jar, or a potato masher, press down as firmly as you can to allow the liquid to rise up and cover the shredded cabbage. You should leave about 1 to 2 inches of space between the cabbage and the top of the jar to give the cabbage room to expand as it ferments. If the mixture has not created enough liquid to cover the cabbage, add enough cool distilled water to completely cover it.

Place a bit of cool water in a small, clean resealable plastic bag, pushing to eliminate all air from the bag. You need just enough water to create a weight to keep the cabbage under the liquid. Seal the bag, place it on top of the cabbage in the jar and push it down to ensure that the water bag has sufficient weight. Place the lid on the container and seal tightly.

Set aside in a cool, dark spot for 5 days. Check the fermentation process daily to make sure the cabbage has remained covered in liquid. If not, add distilled water to cover.

After 2 days, begin tasting the sauerkraut. Remove the water bag and set it aside. Remove and discard any scum or mold that has formed; it is not harmful, just unappetizing. Using a fork, poke around in the jar, and pull out a small amount to taste. This allows you to determine when the sauerkraut is to your liking. But be sure to push the sauerkraut back down into the liquid, place the water bag on top to press the cabbage down, tightly seal, and set aside as before.

Depending on the temperature in its resting place, after one week the sauerkraut should be a bit bubbly and have a tart, sour aroma. When the sauerkraut has reached the flavor and texture you desire, transfer the jar to the refrigerator to impede further fermentation. The kraut will continue to ferment, but at a much slower pace.

You can use the sauerkraut at any point in the fermentation process. Early in the process it will be more cabbage-like and crunchy; later it will be softer and have a stronger, more sour flavor. It will keep, covered and refrigerated, up to six months, although it will slowly continue to increase in sourness.

NOTE: Cabbage ferments very quickly at room temperature (about 70°F), and sauerkraut is usually ready to eat in a week. You can also refrigerate it from the start, but fermentation will occur very slowly (taking somewhat more than double the time of room temperature fermentation); however, the end result will be crisper. If kept at a temperature over 80°F, it will quickly turn dark brown and spoil. If this occurs, discard the sauerkraut and start again.

For more flavor, add caraway, dill, or mustard seeds to the cabbage and salt.

Spiced Asparagus

Makes 1 quart

Asparagus prepared in this manner makes an elegant addition to salads and charcuterie platters, serves as a snappy hors d'oeuvre, and best of all, is good for you! This is a terrific way to preserve that perfect and inexpensive spring harvest.

    1 pound organic asparagus (about 16 spears)
    4 cloves organic garlic, peeled and sliced
    2½ cups room-temperature Spiced Brine (see page 228)

Trim the woody ends from the asparagus. You can then either cut each spear on the bias into 3-inch pieces or neatly trim the end and leave each spear whole.

If using cut pieces, place them in a bowl, add the garlic, and toss to combine. Place into a sterilized 1-quart glass canning jar with a sterilized lid or a 1-quart crock with a sterilized, tight-fitting lid. Pour the brine into the container, taking care that it covers the asparagus completely.

If whole pieces, place the spears, standing with tip up, into a sterilized 1-quart glass canning jar with a sterilized lid or a 1-quart crock with a sterilized, tight-fitting lid. Nestle the garlic slices around the asparagus spears. Pour the brine into the jar, taking care that it covers the asparagus completely.

If there is not enough liquid to cover the asparagus, add enough cool distilled water to completely cover. You should leave about 1 to 2 inches of space between the asparagus and the top of the jar to give the asparagus room to expand as it ferments.

Place a bit of cool water into a small resealable plastic bag, pushing to eliminate all air from the bag. You need just enough water to create a weight to keep the asparagus under the liquid. Seal the bag, and place it on top of the asparagus, pushing down to ensure that the water bag has sufficient weight. Do not press too firmly on the whole spears, as you don't want to smash the tips. Place the lid on the container and seal tightly. Set aside in a cool, dark spot.

Check the jar frequently to make sure the asparagus remains covered with liquid. If the liquid level is low, remove the water bag and set it aside. Remove and discard any scum or mold that has formed (it is not harmful, just unappetizing). Add distilled water to cover the asparagus. Push the asparagus back down into the liquid, place the water bag on top to press the asparagus down, tightly seal, and set aside as before.

After about 1 week the asparagus is ready to eat, but allowing it to ferment for 2 weeks will add more flavor. Transfer to the refrigerator and store for up to 3 months.

Sweet Cippolini Onions

Makes 1 quart

If you can't find small, rather flat white or red cippolini onions, you can use small yellow or red onions or shallots in this recipe. The same goes for the Himalayan pink salt, which is available at specialty food stores, some supermarkets, and online. Other fine sea salts may be used, but they won't add the hint of color to the finished onions that the pink salt does.

Although delicious straight from the jar, a quick turn on the grill heightens the acidic flavor of these pickled onions and makes them the perfect side to a grilled steak or chop.

> 10 whole cloves
>
> 10 cippolini onions, peeled and trimmed (about 1¼ pounds)
>
> 1 one-inch piece fresh ginger root, peeled and sliced
>
> 2 two-inch pieces cinnamon stick
>
> 1 tablespoon fine Himalayan pink salt
>
> Distilled water (about 2 cups—enough to cover the onions)

Stick 1 clove into each onion. Fit half of the onions into a sterilized 1-quart glass canning jar. Nestle half of the ginger around the onions and add the cinnamon sticks. Fit the remaining onions into the jar and nestle the remaining ginger slices around them.

Combine the salt with the water, stirring to dissolve. Pour the salted water over the onions, taking care that it covers them completely. If it doesn't, add enough cool distilled water to completely cover. You should leave about 1 to 2 inches of space between the onions and the top of the jar to give the onions room to expand as they ferment.

Place a bit of cool water into a small resealable plastic bag, pushing to eliminate all air from the bag. You need just enough water to create a weight to keep the onions under the liquid. Seal the bag, and place it on top of the onions, pushing it down to ensure that the water bag has suffi-cient weight. Place a sterilized lid on the container and seal tightly. Set aside in a cool, dark spot for 3 weeks or until the onions are as flavorful as you like.

Check the onions frequently to make sure they remain covered with liquid. If the liquid level is low, remove the water bag and set it aside. Remove and discard any scum or mold that has formed (it is not harmful, just unappetizing). Add distilled water to cover the onions. Push the onions back down into the liquid, place the water bag on top to press them down, tightly seal, and set aside as before.

After 3 weeks the onions should be ready to eat, but another 2 weeks of fermentation at room temperature will not hurt them. Transfer to the refrigerator and store for up to 9 months.

Kimchi

Makes 1 quart

Kimchi is one of those traditional recipes for which every Korean home cook has a secret or long-handed-down recipe. Traditionally, it was pre-pared in glazed clay crocks and buried deep in the ground to ripen over long periods of time, but that is rarely done anymore.

Fresh kimchi is treated as a salad; when ripened, it is used as a side dish or condiment; and when really mature, it is only for the stouthearted, as it is quite sour and intensely flavored. It is a dish you can make your own by adding more heat or changing the vegetables used. However, no matter what combination you choose, make sure you keep the pear or apple, as their sugars assist in the fermentation.

I recommend that you weigh the cabbage after you have removed the core and any wilted or damaged outer leaves.

2 pounds organic napa or savoy cabbage, cut into pieces about 2-inches square

¼ cup plus 1 tablespoon fine pure sea salt

¼ cup gochugaru or pure organic hot chili powder (see note)

1 large organic Asian pear, bosc pear, or crisp apple, skin-on, cored and chopped

2 tablespoons chopped organic garlic

1 tablespoon minced organic ginger root

1 tablespoon natural anchovy paste

2 organic leeks, white and some green parts, well washed and chopped

1 large organic Japanese radish (daikon), trimmed and cut into matchsticks

1 organic carrot, trimmed and cut into matchsticks

1 raw organic chicory (endive) root, well washed, peeled, and cut into matchsticks (optional—see note)

½ cup (about 3 ounces) chopped organic Jerusalem artichokes

Combine the cabbage with ¼ cup of the salt in a large mixing bowl. Add enough warm distilled water to cover. Using your hands, mix the cabbage into the salted water. Set aside, uncovered, for 4 to 8 hours.

Drain the salted cabbage into a colander, and rinse under cold running water, shaking off excess water. Place the cabbage in a large mixing bowl.

Combine the gochugaru with the pear, garlic, ginger, and anchovy paste in a food processor fitted with a metal blade. Add 1 cup of warm distilled water, and process to a smooth puree. Set aside.

Toss the leeks, radish, carrot, chicory root, and Jerusalem artichokes into the cabbage. Using a rubber spatula, scrape the chile puree into the vegetables. Put on rubber gloves (to prevent the chiles from burning your skin), and use your hands to thoroughly rub the chile paste and the remaining salt into the vegetables.

Still wearing the gloves, pack the mixture and the liquid it has formed into a sterilized container, such as a 1-quart glass canning jar with a sterilized lid or a 1-quart crock with a sterilized, tight-fitting lid. Using your gloved fingertips, a smaller jar or glass that will fit down into the larger jar, or a potato masher, press down as firmly as you can so the liquid rises up and covers the vegetables. If the mixture has not created enough liquid to cover, add cool distilled water to completely cover. You should leave about 1 to 2 inches of space between the vegetables and the top of the jar to give the kimchi room to expand as it ferments.

Place a bit of cool water into a small resealable plastic bag, pushing to eliminate all air from the bag. You need just enough water to create a weight to keep the vegetables under the liquid. Seal the bag and place it on top of the kimchi, pushing it down to ensure that the water bag has sufficient weight. Place the lid on the container and seal tightly.

Set aside in a cool, dark spot for 3 days. Check the kimchi daily to make sure it remains covered with liquid. If not, add distilled water to cover.

It is said that the optimal length of time for kimchi fermentation is three days, but many cooks allow it to ferment for far longer periods. It really depends on how sour and/or zesty you want it to be. After 3 days, begin tasting the kimchi to see if it is as flavorful as you'd like. Place the water bag back on top, reseal, and set aside as before.

When the kimchi has reached the flavor you desire, transfer the jar to the refrigerator to impede the fermentation process. The kimchi will continue to ferment, but at a much slower pace.

NOTE: Gochugaru, an essential ingredient in Korean cooking, is simply dried and crushed Korean red chiles. It is coarsely textured, a deep and pulsating red, and very spicy with a soft sweet aftertone. There is no replacement for it in authentic Korean cooking. The closest thing would be to grind your own dried organic hot red chiles. You should only purchase gochugaru made from 100% pure Korean red chiles; however, if you can't find it, use pure organic chili powder.

I use chicory root, as it is an excellent source of antioxidants as well as a terrific system cleanser. But since it is not always easy to find, I have made it optional; it will not impact the flavor or texture of the finished kimchi.

MEAT, FISH, AND EGGS

Corned Beef

Makes 6–8 pounds

This is traditionally served with plain cooked cabbage. However, to maximize brain-making potential, I serve my corned beef with home-made sauerkraut (see page 236). A large cut of beef will take approximately 2 weeks to ferment; thinner cuts, such as brisket, will be corned in about 5 days.

6 quarts Spiced Brine (see page 228)

2 cups raw honey

1 six- to eight-pound grass-fed beef top round roast

12 organic black peppercorns

6 sprigs organic parsley

4 bay leaves

3 cloves organic garlic, peeled and chopped

Distilled water for cooking

6 organic leeks with some green part, trimmed and well washed

4 carrots, peeled and cut into chunks

Sauerkraut (optional)

Hot mustard (optional)

Combine the brine and the honey in a large saucepan over high heat and bring to a boil. Lower the heat and cook at a gentle simmer for about 5 minutes or just until the honey has dissolved. Remove from the heat and set aside to cool.

Place the beef into the cooled brine, making sure that it is completely covered by the brine. If not, add enough cold distilled water to cover. Cover and refrigerate for up to 2 weeks, checking often to ensure the meat is completely covered. After 1 week, begin checking to see how deeply the brine flavor has been imparted to the meat. Remove the meat from the liquid and slice off a thin end piece. Quickly sear the piece just enough to allow you to taste it. You want the pickled flavor to be dominant without being too salty. If a deeper pickled flavor is desired, return the meat to the brine, cover, and refrigerate for the additional week, again checking often to ensure the meat is completely covered and doing the taste test every other day.

When ready to cook, remove the meat from the brine, and discard the brine.

Combine the peppercorns, parsley, bay leaves, and garlic in a small piece of cheesecloth. Using kitchen twine, tie the cheesecloth into a little bag. Set aside.

Place the meat in a large Dutch oven. Add cold distilled water to cover. Add the cheesecloth bag along with the leeks and carrots. Place over high heat and bring to a boil. Lower the heat and cook at a gentle simmer—adding more distilled water if needed to keep the meat submerged—for about 3 hours or until the meat is tender when pierced with the point of a small sharp knife.

Remove the beef from the liquid and cut it, against the grain, into thin slices. Place the slices on a serving platter along with the leeks. Serve with sauerkraut and hot mustard, if desired.

Corned Spiced Pork Loin

Makes 4 pounds

Lean pork loin works best for brining, as pork fat often does not taste good or look appetizing when brined. Although delicious hot with sauerkraut, this spiced pork loin is a tasty addition to a chef's salad, stir fries, or soups.

3 quarts plus 1 cup distilled water

¾ cup fine pure sea salt

1 tablespoon organic brown sugar

6 bay leaves

5 whole star anise

1 cinnamon stick

1 teaspoon mustard seeds

1 teaspoon juniper berries

1 teaspoon whole coriander

1 teaspoon whole allspice

½ teaspoon red chili flakes

¼ cup coarse salt, preferably Himalayan pink salt

4 pounds pork loin, trimmed of all excess fat

4 cloves garlic, peeled and halved lengthwise

6 cups Sauerkraut (see page 236)

2 cups thinly sliced onion

Hot mustard or horseradish (optional)

Combine the 3 quarts of water with the sea salt and sugar in a large, non-reactive saucepan, stirring to dissolve. Place over high heat, and add the bay leaves, star anise, cinnamon stick, mustard seeds, juniper berries, coriander, allspice, and chili flakes. Bring to a boil, and boil for 5 minutes. Remove from the heat, add the coarse salt, and set aside to cool.

Place the pork and garlic in a large resealable plastic bag (use 2-gallon storage bags or brining bags). Pour the cooled brine into the bag, push out the air, and seal. Place the bag in a container large enough to hold the pork in a position that will ensure that it remains covered with the brine. Transfer to the refrigerator, and allow it to brine for 1 week, checking often to make sure the meat is completely covered with brine.

Remove from the refrigerator, drain, and discard the brine.

Place the meat in a Dutch oven. Add the sauerkraut and sliced onion, along with the remaining cup of distilled water. Place over high heat, and bring to a boil. Immediately lower the heat, cover, and simmer for about 90 minutes or until the meat is tender when pierced with the point of a small sharp knife.

Transfer the meat to a cutting board. Using a sharp chef's knife, cut it crosswise into thin slices. Lay the slices, slightly overlapping, down the center of a serving platter. Spoon the sauerkraut/onion mixture around the edge of the platter, and serve with hot mustard on the side, if desired.

Pickled Sardines

Makes 1½ pounds

This recipe is based on the classic Swedish pickled herring, but I have used nutrient-rich sardines in place of the traditional herring. You can, of course, use herring or some other small fish, such as whitebait or smelt.

1½ pounds wild sardine fillets

Approximately 4 cups room temperature Spiced Brine
  (see page 228)

1 cup distilled water

2 cups raw vinegar

¼ cup raw honey

3 bay leaves

3 whole cloves

1 organic sweet onion, peeled and cut crosswise into thin slices

1 organic Meyer lemon, cut crosswise into thin slices

Place the fillets in a shallow container. Add enough brine to completely cover the fish. Cover the entire container with plastic film, and refrigerate for 24 hours.

Combine the distilled water with the vinegar and honey in a small saucepan over medium heat. Bring to a boil, then lower the heat and cook at a bare simmer for 5 minutes. Remove from the heat and let cool.

Remove the sardines from the refrigerator. Uncover and pour off the brine. Place the fillets in a clean, sterilized container, such as a 1-quart glass canning jar with a sterilized lid, and randomly add the bay leaves, cloves, and onion and lemon slices as you fill the jar. Add the cooled vinegar mixture. If the fish is not covered completely, add enough cool distilled water to cover. You should leave about 1 to 2 inches of space between the fish and the top of the jar to allow the gases to be released as the fish ferments. Let stand at room temperature for 24 hours; transfer to the refrigerator for 1 day before eating. May be stored, covered and refrigerated, for up to 1 month.

NOTE: To make Creamed Pickled Sardines, remove the sardines from the pickling liquid at the end of the pickling process, reserving ¼ cup of the liquid. Place the sardines in a serving bowl. Combine the reserved liquid with 1 cup Quark (see page 233), whisking to blend well, and pour the mixture over the sardines. Add 2 thinly sliced sweet onions and a tablespoon of chopped fresh dill and toss to blend. Cover and refrigerate for at least 1 hour to allow flavors to blend. Serve, or store—covered and refrigerated—for up to 2 weeks.

Scandinavian-Style Fermented Salmon

Makes 2 pounds

Although many Scandinavian fermented fish recipes result in strongly flavored dishes that are an acquired taste, this one creates a citrusy flavor that is much more appealing to the American palate. This salmon makes a wonderful passed hors d'oeuvre or a terrific topping for a mixed green or vegetable salad.

> Approximately 3 cups room temperature Spiced Brine (see page 228)
>
> ¼ cup room temperature Whey (see page 225)
>
> 1 tablespoon raw honey
>
> 2 pounds boneless, skinless wild salmon, cut into bite-size pieces
>
> 6 sprigs fresh organic dill
>
> 1 whole organic lemon, cut crosswise into thin slices

Combine the brine with the whey and honey, stirring to blend well.

Place the fish pieces in a clean, sterilized container, such as a 1-quart glass canning jar with a sterilized lid, randomly adding the dill sprigs and lemon slices as you fill the jar. Add the brine mixture. If the fish is not covered completely, add enough cool distilled water to cover. You should leave about 1 to 2 inches of space between the fish and the top of the jar to allow the gases to be released as the fish ferments. Let stand at room temperature for 24 hours; transfer to the refrigerator at least 4 hours or up to 1 week before serving.

Raw Fish Ferment

Makes 1½ pounds

This recipe is much like sushi from generations past when it was made with salted, fermented fish rather than the raw fish with which we are now familiar. Unlike many other strong-smelling fish dishes that are fermented for longer periods, this brief cure creates a mellow dish that still offers the digestive aid and nutritional value of longer ferments.

I have made this recipe with both whey and sauerkraut juice and find that although both work, the sauerkraut juice offers the best flavor.

1½ pounds wild fish fillets, cut into bite-size pieces

5 thin slices peeled organic ginger root

1 organic onion, peeled and chopped

Approximately 1½ cups sauerkraut juice, homemade (see page 236) or commercially produced

Place the fish in a clean, sterilized container, such as a 1-quart glass canning jar with a sterilized lid, randomly adding the ginger and onion pieces as you fill the jar. Add the sauerkraut juice. If the fish is not covered completely, add enough cool distilled water to cover. You should leave about 1 to 2 inches of space between the fish and the top of the jar to allow the gases to be released as the fish ferments. Let stand at room temperature for 8 hours; transfer to the refrigerator to cure for no more than 3 days.

Once chilled, the fish may be eaten plain or with a drizzle of extra-virgin olive oil, lemon juice, and sea salt.

Fermented Hard-Boiled Eggs

Makes 1 dozen

These pickled eggs make a terrific snack or an addition to a salad. You can also use the Spiced Brine (see page 228) for the ferment to add some more flavor.

1 dozen hard-boiled eggs, peeled

6 cloves organic garlic, peeled and halved lengthwise

3 sprigs organic dill

3 organic dried red hot chiles

¼ cup room temperature Whey (see page 225)

Approximately 2 cups room temperature Basic Brine (see page 227)

Place about three of the eggs in the bottom of a clean, sterilized container, such as a 1-quart canning jar with a sterilized lid or a crock with a sterilized, tight-fitting lid. Randomly add garlic, dill, and chiles as you continue adding eggs to fill the container. Add the whey followed by enough brine to cover the eggs. You should leave about 1 to 2 inches of space between the eggs and the top of the jar to allow the gases to be released as the eggs ferment. Cover tightly and set aside in a cool, dark spot for 3 days. Because the eggs have been cooked, there will not be a large amount of gaseous bubbling; expect to see just slight bubbling on the top when fermentation is complete. Once fermentation has occurred, transfer to the refrigerator for up to 3 weeks.

FRUITS

Preserved Lemons

Makes 1 pint

Preserved lemons are an essential ingredient in Moroccan cooking. They are used to season salads, tagines, and grain dishes. I like them chopped in salads and stews, sliced with grilled fish, and mixed with herbs to season a roast chicken. They are easy to make and keep forever.

Working with one at a time, place the lemons on a flat surface and roll them around, pressing down lightly to soften. Do not press too hard or the lemons will split and be unusable.

Cut each lemon in half crosswise, and then cut each half, lengthwise, into four equal pieces without cutting all the way through. You want the lemon to open slightly like a blooming flower. Remove and discard any seeds.

Place some salt in the crevices of each lemon. Then, using a small portion of the remaining salt, place a thin layer of salt in the bottom of a clean, sterilized pint container, such as a 1-pint glass canning jar with a sterilized lid or a 1-pint crock with a sterilized, tight-fitting lid. The container should be barely large enough to hold the lemons, as it is essential that they be very tightly packed. Begin tightly packing the lemons into the container, following each layer of lemons with another layer of salt. Continue packing in the lemon pieces until all of the lemons and salt have been used. As you pack, you will compress the lemons, and they will begin to exude a lot of juice. If using cinnamon sticks, randomly place them among the lemons. If the lemons have not exuded enough juice to cover them completely, add additional lemon juice to cover. You should leave about 1 inch of space between the lemons and the top of the jar to give them room to expand as they ferment.

Place a bit of cool water into a small resealable plastic bag, pushing to eliminate all air from the bag. You need just enough water to create a weight to keep the lemons under the liquid. Seal the bag, and place it on top of the lemons, pushing down to ensure that the water bag has sufficient weight.

Place the lid on the container and seal tightly. Let the lemons ferment at room temperature for 1 week, checking the container frequently to make sure the lemons remain covered with liquid. If the liquid level is low, using some force, push the lemons down so the liquid can rise up to cover them. Place the water bag back on top to press them down, tightly seal, and set aside at room temperature for at least 2 more weeks before using.

Preserved lemons may be stored at room temperature for up to 1 year. Throughout the fermentation, remove and discard any scum or mold that forms (it is not harmful, just unappetizing). The lemons may also be stored, covered and refrigerated, for an even longer period.

NOTE: Although most organic lemons have not been waxed, if you have any question about yours, blanch them in boiling water for 1 minute before using. Drain well and set aside to cool completely before proceeding with the recipe.

Blueberry-Mint Preserves

Makes 1 pint

These are far different from highly sweetened commercial jams. The honey does add some mellow, sugary taste, but the fermentation and the whey add quite a strong note of acidity. You can use any berry except strawberries (which don't seem to "jell" during fermentation) and any herb or spice you like to make this jam your own.

3 cups organic blueberries

⅓ cup raw honey

1 teaspoon fine pure sea salt

2 tablespoons chopped fresh organic mint leaves

1 teaspoon organic lemon juice

¼ cup Whey (see page 225) or vegan starter (see Resources)

Combine 2½ cups of the berries with the honey and salt in a medium saucepan over medium heat. Bring to a low simmer, and begin mashing the berries with the back of a wooden spoon. Simmer for 5 minutes. Remove from the heat, and set aside to cool.

Combine the remaining ½ cup blueberries with the mint leaves and lemon juice in a food processor fitted with a metal blade. Process for about 1 minute or until pureed. Pour the puree into the cooled berry mixture. Add the whey, stirring to blend well.

Pour the mixture into clean containers, such as two sterilized 8-ounce glass jelly canning jars with sterilized lids or two ½-pint crocks with sterilized, tight-fitting lids. Cover tightly, and set aside at room temperature for 2 days to allow fermentation. The preserves may be consumed immediately. Once opened, they may be stored in the refrigerator for up to 1 month or the freezer for up to 3 months.

CONDIMENTS

Jicama Pickle

Makes about 1 quart

Jicama is one of the top probiotic foods. Jerusalem artichoke may also be used in this recipe. These pickles are simple to make and terrific to keep on hand for snacking or salads. You can change the flavor by using other herbs, adding some spices or chiles, or using lemon or lime peel in place of the orange.

1 large organic orange (see note)
1¼ pounds organic jicama, peeled and cut into 1-inch cubes
6 sprigs fresh organic dill
6 sprigs fresh organic mint
2 cups room temperature Basic Brine (see page 227)

Using a small, sharp knife, remove the peel from the orange, taking care that no white pith is attached. Place half of the peel in the bottom of a sterilized container, such as a 1-quart glass canning jar with a sterilized lid or a 1-quart crock with a sterilized, tight-fitting lid. Add half of the jicama along with half of the dill and mint. Then make another layer of orange peel, jicama, dill, and mint. Pour the brine into the container. You should leave about 1 to 2 inches of space between the jicama and the top of the jar to give it room to expand as it ferments.

Place a bit of cool water into a small resealable plastic bag, pushing to eliminate all air from the bag. You need just enough water to create a weight to keep the jicama under the liquid. Seal the bag, and place it on top of the jicama, pushing down to ensure that the water bag has sufficient weight. Place the lid on the container and seal tightly.

Set aside to ferment at room temperature in a cool, dark spot for 3 days. Check the container daily to make sure the jicama remains covered with liquid. If not, add cool distilled water to cover.

After 3 days, open the container. Remove the water bag and set it aside. Remove and discard the herbs. This can be a bit messy, but if you leave the herbs in for a longer period, they will deteriorate and get a bit mushy.

Push the jicama back down into the liquid, place the water bag back on top to press the jicama down, tightly seal, and set aside as before. Check daily to test for flavor and texture. Depending on the temperature in the dark spot you've chosen, the jicama should be ready to eat after 10 days. When it has reached the flavor and texture you desire, transfer the jar to the refrigerator to impede the fermentation process. The jicama may be stored, covered and refrigerated, for up to 6 weeks.

NOTE: Although most organic citrus has not been waxed, if you have any question about yours, blanch it in boiling water for 1 minute before using. Drain well and set aside to cool completely before proceeding with the recipe.

Pickled Garlic

Makes about 2 cups

These zesty cloves are a great addition to so many things and even make a tasty pop-in-your-mouth snack. Pickled garlic can brighten salads, hummus, soups, or stews and can make an inviting cocktail tidbit stuck on a toothpick with a piece of rare grass-fed beef.

> 50 cloves (about 4 heads) garlic, peeled and trimmed of any brown spots
>
> 2 cups room temperature Basic Brine (see page 227)

Place the garlic in a clean, sterilized container, such as a 1-quart glass canning jar with a sterilized lid. Add the brine, taking care that it covers the garlic completely. If not, add just enough cool distilled water to cover.

Place a bit of cool water into a small resealable plastic bag, pushing to eliminate all air from the bag. You need just enough water to create a weight to keep the garlic under the liquid. Seal the bag, and place it on top of the garlic, pushing down to ensure that the water bag has sufficient weight. Place the lid on the container and seal tightly.

Set aside at room temperature in a cool, dark spot for 1 month. Check the container after 2 weeks to ensure that the brine still covers the garlic. If it does not, add more brine to cover.

The garlic is usually ready to eat after 1 month, by which time the strong, raw aroma is replaced by a slightly sweet one. From time to time throughout the month, do a taste test; continue fermenting until the texture and taste are to your liking.

Pickled garlic keeps, covered and refrigerated, almost indefinitely.

Pickled Salsa

Makes about 2 pints

Since I am not a chip eater, I use this salsa as a sauce for grilled meats and fish. It is particularly delicious in a shellfish cocktail in place of the usual cocktail sauce. It also makes a great lunch when stirred into a bowl of homemade yogurt.

2 cups diced, peeled, and seeded organic tomatoes

1 cup diced organic red onion

1 cup diced jicama

½ cup chopped organic cilantro

1 tablespoon minced organic garlic

1 tablespoon minced organic hot chili, or to taste

Juice of 1 organic lime, plus more to taste

3 tablespoons Whey (see page 225)

1 teaspoon fine pure sea salt, or more to taste

Combine the tomatoes, onion, jicama, cilantro, garlic, and chili in a large nonreactive bowl. Stir in the lime juice, whey, and salt. Taste and, if necessary, add additional lime juice or salt.

Spoon equal portions of the salsa into each of three clean, sterilized containers, such as 1-pint glass canning jars with sterilized lids. You should leave about 1 to 2 inches of space between the salsa and the top of the jar to give the mixture room to expand as it ferments. Place the lid on the container and seal tightly.

Set aside at room temperature in a cool, dark spot for up to 3 days or just until the salsa has the flavor and texture you prefer. Transfer to the refrigerator and store, covered and refrigerated, for up to 3 months.

BEVERAGES

Kombucha

Makes 3 quarts

Kombucha, a traditional drink in Asian cultures, has only recently been discovered in America. It is known to be a very strong detoxifier and is loaded with vitamins and amino acids. Although it can be purchased in health food stores and some supermarkets, there is nothing better than a homemade batch.

To make kombucha, you will need a large (about 1 gallon) glass container, a clean cloth, and what is known as a SCOBY (Symbiotic Colony of Bacteria and Yeast), which is available from most health food stores or online (see Resources). The SCOBY is often referred to as the "mother" or the "mushroom" of kombucha; the former because it is the source of the drink's life, and the latter because when it forms in the drink it resembles a large flaccid fungus. All in all, kombucha can look a bit foreboding, with the SCOBY seeming to take on the appearance of all kinds of faces, from pimply to stringy to just plain weird. However, these looks do not affect the taste unless mold appears. If any black or blue mold does appear on the SCOBY, discard both it and the tea immediately. Sterilize your container, and start all over again.

3 quarts distilled water

1 cup unrefined sugar

6 bags organic green tea

1 SCOBY (see note 1)

1 cup fermented kombucha or raw cider vinegar, such as Bragg's (see note 2)

Place the water in a large saucepan over high heat. Add the sugar and bring to a boil. Boil for 5 minutes, and then add the tea bags. Remove from the heat and set aside for 15 minutes to steep.

After steeping, remove and discard the tea bags. Allow the tea to cool to room temperature.

When cool, transfer the tea to a sterilized 1-gallon glass jar. Add the SCOBY with the shiny surface facing up. Add the fermented kombucha or vinegar. The SCOBY might sink, but it will rise again during fermentation. (If, for any reason, you feel the need to lift or move it, use a clean wooden spoon; metal does not react well with a SCOBY.)

Cover the container with a clean cloth and secure the cloth in place with a large rubber band. The cloth simply keeps dust, airborne spores, and insects from contaminating the drink.

Set the jar aside to ferment at room temperature (no less than 65°F and no more than 90°F) in a dark spot for 5 to 10 days. The temperature is important because if it is too cool the drink will take too long to ferment. Begin testing for taste after the fourth day. The tea should not be too sweet; if it is, the sugar has not yet been converted. Perfectly brewed kombucha should have a fizzy tartness that most resembles sparkling cider. If it becomes too acidic or has a very vinegary odor, it has fermented for too long. It is drinkable but not as tasty as it should be.

When the kombucha is nicely carbonated and as flavorful as you desire, pour it into sterilized glass containers, seal, and refrigerate. Discard the SCOBY. The kombucha will keep, covered and refrigerated, for up to 1 year.

NOTE 1: Both the SCOBY and fermented kombucha are available from health food stores and online. Although raw vinegar can replace the fermented kombucha, I suggest beginning your kombucha-making with fermented kombucha as it will absolutely guarantee that you will create a successful batch, whereas raw vinegar does not give you this guarantee.

NOTE 2: Certified Bragg Organic Raw Apple Cider Vinegar is available from health food stores, specialty food stores, many supermarkets, and online. It is unfiltered, unheated, and unpasteurized, with 5% acidity.

Water Kefir

Makes 1 quart

Unlike milk-based kefir, water kefir is a probiotic beverage made with sugared or coconut water or juice and flavored with juice, pure extracts, or dried fruit. Kefir grains or powdered kefir starter culture are required to activate the fermentation. Kefir "grains" are composed of bacteria and yeast working together in a symbiotic relationship but do not contain actual wheat (or other) grain; the term is used to describe their look.

4 cups warm distilled water

¼ cup unrefined sugar

3 teaspoons water kefir grains (see note and Resources)

¼ cup organic blueberry (or any other organic fruit) juice

Pour the water into a large (slightly more than 1 quart) sterilized glass jar, taking care to leave at least 1 inch of space between the water and the top of the jar so there is room for the pressure to build as the drink ferments.

Add the sugar to the water, stirring occasionally until the sugar has dissolved and the water has cooled. Do not add the kefir grains until the water is cool; they will not activate properly in warm water.

When the water is cool, add the kefir grains. Cover the container with a clean cloth, and secure the cloth in place with a large rubber band. The cloth simply keeps dust, airborne spores, and insects from contaminating the drink.

Set aside to ferment at room temperature. Check on the progress of the fermentation after 24 hours. Do not allow the fermentation to continue beyond 2 days. After 2 days, the fermentation might kill the kefir grains. When it is ready, the kefir will be rather sweet, but not as sweet as the sugar water base; it may also be slightly carbonated. Although it can now be consumed, a second fermentation (described below) will give it more flavor.

Strain the liquid through a nonreactive strainer into a 1-quart sterilized glass container with a sterilized, tight-fitting lid, reserving the kefir grains. The grains may be stored for reuse; if you wish to do so, store them, covered and refrigerated, in the same amount of sugar and water that is used in this recipe.

Add the blueberry juice to the water kefir, taking care to leave at least 1 inch of space between the flavored water and the top of the jar so that pressure can build as the drink ferments. Cover tightly and set aside at room temperature (no less than 65°F and no more than 90°F) in a dark spot for up to 2 days. The temperature is important because if it is too hot the beverage will ferment too quickly, and if it is too cool fermentation will take too long. Transfer to the refrigerator, and let the kefir rest for 3 days to allow the carbonation to set.

When it is ready to drink, open the jar carefully, as the kefir might foam up and out of the bottle due to the pressure that has built up.

NOTE: Water kefir grains differ from milk kefir grains and are generally used to make kefirs based on fruit juices or sugared waters. Water kefir grains (also known as *tibicos*) are a SCOBY, a Symbiotic Colony of Bacteria and Yeast. Water kefir grains are used only for culturing water kefir; they proliferate best in a high-mineral environment, such as that provided by unrefined organic cane sugar. Water kefir cannot be made with milk kefir grains because milk kefir grains are composed of different beneficial bacteria and yeasts that are dependent upon milk to grow and reproduce. Although you can use milk kefir grains to culture nondairy liquids (such as coconut water), they must be returned to milk for storage to ensure that they retain their strength.

Coconut Water Lemonade

Makes about 4½ cups

This refreshing drink is very good for you. Although I make it with coconut water, you can also use distilled water.

    4 cups organic coconut water
    ¼ cup plus 1 tablespoon unrefined sugar
    4 sprigs fresh mint
    2 tablespoons water kefir grains (see Resources)
    ⅓ cup fresh organic lemon juice

Combine ½ cup of the coconut water with ¼ cup of the sugar and mint in a small saucepan over medium heat. Cook, stirring frequently, for about 3 minutes or just until the sugar has dissolved. Remove from the heat and set aside to cool.

When it is cool, remove and discard the mint sprigs. Combine the cooled sugared coconut water with the remaining 3½ cups coconut water and the kefir grains in a large (slightly more than 1 quart) sterilized glass container with a sterilized, tight-fitting lid. Cover tightly and set aside at room temperature in a dark spot for 2 days.

Strain the liquid through a nonreactive strainer into a sterilized glass container with a sterilized, tight-fitting lid, reserving the kefir grains. The kefir grains may be stored for reuse; if you wish to do so, store them, covered and refrigerated, in the same amount of sugar and water that is used in this recipe.

Combine the lemon juice with the remaining 1 tablespoon of sugar, stirring to dissolve.

Add the lemon juice mixture to the coconut water kefir, taking care to leave at least 1 inch of space between the kefir and the top of the jar so that pressure can build as the drink ferments. Cover tightly and set aside at room temperature in a dark spot for up to 1 day. (If it is allowed to ferment for more than 1 day, the process can produce so much carbonation that the liquid might explode out of the bottle when it is opened.) Transfer to the refrigerator and chill for at least 4 hours before serving.

When it is ready to drink, open carefully as the lemonade might foam up and out of the bottle due to the pressure that has built up. If it does not taste sweet enough, add a bit of stevia.

What the Future Holds

ON ANY GIVEN DAY WHEN I have a chance to tune out my work responsibilities and enjoy some R&R (another must for nurturing the microbiome!), I'm often out at sea on my boat fishing or camping under the stars. I commune with Mother Nature on a regular basis. I know of her kindness and beauty, and from my professional life I understand her wrath as well.

In the last century, it seems we've tried to shut nature out in a lot of ways, believing that it harbors germs and deadly pathogens. After Alexander Fleming discovered penicillin, we as a society got stuck on the germ theory of disease. In Dr. David B. Agus's seminal book *The End of Illness*, he writes:[1]

> We've had a hard time moving past the germ theory of disease, which dominated, and in many ways defined, medicine in the twentieth century. According to this theory, if you can figure out what species of germ you are infected with, then your problem is solved because that tells you how you should treat the disease. This became the general paradigm of medicine.... The treatment only cared about the invading organism, such as the bacterium that causes tuberculosis or the parasite that leads to malaria;

it didn't care to define or understand the host (the human being) or even where the infection was happening in the host....

Indeed, understanding the human host is fundamental. If we hope to make headway in improving our health, we can no longer rely on thinking that what ails us can be blamed squarely on a single germ or even a single genetic mutation. The chronic conditions of today, especially those that end up crippling or disabling the neurological system and brain, are diseases of the body's entire system. And that system, to be sure, includes the microbiome.

Dr. Agus goes on to highlight a most interesting historical note in his book. No sooner did the germ theory of disease explode as antibiotics were being discovered than renowned geneticist J. B. S. Haldane warned people during a talk at Cambridge in 1923 that focusing on pathogenic germs would lead us astray in understanding human physiology. In fact, he made an unforgettable prediction: "This is a disaster for medicine because we're going to get focused on these germs, and we're going to forget about the system." That system—the human body—is no doubt largely dominated by, controlled by, defined by, comprised of, and orchestrated by the gut's microbial residents. Although he was speaking almost one hundred years ago, Haldane was spot on. His sentiments were later echoed by Dr. Fleming himself, the man who discovered the first antibiotic.

Unfortunately, we as a society have reached a place where we reflexively seek culprits to blame for our health challenges. And we assume that they originate from the outside world. To some degree, that is true in terms of the foods and chemicals we bring into our bodies. But it's categorically wrong to think our modern afflictions arise from external germs. The germ theory is useless for trying to understand conditions like obesity, cancer, dementia, and mysterious autoimmune diseases. Our health woes stem from what's going on *inside*. And not only will our cures in the future address this fact with new technologies to treat the system as a whole, but they will also likely rely on our microbial collaborators.

Throughout this book I have mentioned one such technology currently in development: fecal microbial transplantation (FMT). I think this one in particular is poised to stir a revolution in medicine and finally arm doctors with an effective way to treat some of our most challenging disorders—from autoimmune diseases to grave neurological disorders. Let's take a look at one woman's story so you can grasp the power and promise of FMT.

MANY SYMPTOMS, NO DIAGNOSIS, BUT A SINGLE SOLUTION

Fifty-four-year-old Margaret, who, ironically, owns and operates a health food store, came to see me because of generalized fatigue, brain fog, body aches, and essentially being unable to carry on with her life. She had endured this miserable state of being for ten long years. Problems began after she returned from a trip to the Amazon, after which she developed an infection of unknown origin characterized by coughing and fever. She was prescribed several rounds of antibiotics, but they didn't do the trick. She remained ill for the next year despite being evaluated by several infectious disease specialists at both the esteemed Mayo and Cleveland Clinics.

Nothing specific was found—no smoking gun or invading germ. Soon after these tests failed to reveal any definitive diagnosis, she was hospitalized with another infection in her lungs. She told me that during this time she would experience the sudden onset of nausea, instability, disorientation, and the sense that her "body was feeling heavy, along with sweats." These symptoms recurred regularly every few months after her hospitalization. Eventually, she went to see a neurologist who performed an intensive workup that included an evaluation for seizures. Again, every test was a dead end; nothing was found. Margaret once again landed in the hospital, this time for colitis—a bowel infection— and began receiving intravenous and then oral antibiotics.

In sharing her medical history, she said that she'd had a lifelong exposure to antibiotics for all kinds of problems, including ear infections, throat infections, and respiratory infections, as well as for various surgical issues, including a total hysterectomy, repair of a hernia, and an abdominal infection. She said that her digestive system had been "slow" all her life. At the time of our visit, she was chronically constipated, and her abdomen would become severely bloated immediately after eating. In fact, because of these complaints, she was currently taking high-dosage antibiotics in an attempt to reduce the number of pathogenic, gas-producing bacteria in her small intestine. While the prescribing doctor may have been on to something when he aimed to change her gut's bacteria, he likely wasn't considering the health of her gut's microbiome in its entirety, and he was making matters worse by suggesting that antibiotics would help.

For me, the picture was crystal clear. Here was a woman who had experienced an overwhelming series of medical events that had radically altered her gut microbiome. Margaret herself stated at one point: "My life has been just one antibiotic after another." And evidently this had been going on since her early childhood.

At first I treated her with probiotics and noted some slight improvement. It became evident, however, that just giving her probiotics and modifying her diet was not going to be enough to reverse the negative effects from a lifelong exposure to antibiotics. So we decided to jump in with both feet, and I arranged for her to undergo a fecal transplant, the most aggressive therapy one can take to reset and recolonize a very sick microbiome. (Again, for the record: I myself do not perform the fecal transplant procedure. And the reason my patients often go outside of the U.S. to receive this treatment—or they perform this procedure at home—is because it's not readily available here in the U.S. except for the treatment of a recurring *C. difficile* infection, though I trust this will change very soon. The FDA is currently in the midst of trying to determine how to regulate this procedure, especially for treating illnesses beyond C. *difficile* infections. This makes sense given that the procedure does involve the transfer of bodily fluids from one individual to another and could represent a health threat. It's imperative for donors to be screened for things like HIV and hepatitis and even for dangerous parasites. Clinics in Europe that have been performing these procedures for decades do just that.)

Margaret received one implant each morning for six days. Three months later, the time it took for her microbiome to recolonize, her words captured the improvements:

> For the first time in my life I have regular bowel movements every morning without fail. No more bloating and no more brain fog, headaches, and depression. My whole life, I felt my gut and brain were hijacked...and no physician could figure out why. Well, I finally got the control back and I'm starting to navigate with hope and a feeling of health for the first time in my life. That's an enormous big deal for me, because I was about done with it all.

SH*T FOR BRAINS

These days, we have become accustomed to the notion of replacing a sick or damaged body part with a more functional part from a normal or healthy individual. Whether it's a heart, kidney, or even bone marrow transplant, the idea of a transplant is certainly something that has gained acceptance in modern medicine. But what about people with a damaged, dysfunctional microbiome? What can we offer them besides dietary and lifestyle changes, and perhaps aggressive probiotics treatment?

If the human microbiome is looked upon as an organ, then the notion of transplanting one from a healthy individual to an individual with a damaged microbiome should be embraced. To be clear, this form of transplantation basically means harvesting the fecal material from a healthy individual and "transplanting" that fecal material into the colon of another individual by colonoscopy, endoscopy, sigmoidoscopy, or enema. Right off the bat there's a strong "ick factor" associated with even thinking about transplanting someone's poop into another individual. But when you consider the health consequences of an altered gut microbiome, this may in the future prove to be among the most powerful medical interventions ever devised. And I trust that we'll find other ways of performing this procedure to take the repugnance out of it.

In fact, in October 2014, news of this transplant in pill form took the media by storm. Here's the gist of what a new study, conducted by a team at Harvard Medical School, Massachusetts General Hospital, and Boston Children's Hospital and published in JAMA, revealed: Twenty patients with C. *difficile* received a series of pills filled with frozen bacteria from healthy donors.[2] The researchers made the pills by mixing stool with saline, filtering the solution, extracting the bacteria, transferring the bacteria into pills, and then freezing them. Over the course of two days, each patient swallowed a total of 30 pills. Fully 90 percent of the patients experienced an end to their diarrhea, most within a matter of days following treatment. Although this wasn't the first time researchers have tried to put poop-derived gut bacteria into a pill, this was the first study, albeit a small one, to show how effective oral fecal transplants could be.

The first formally published report of a fecal transplant for medical purposes appeared in the journal *Surgery* in 1958. The procedure was used as a heroic measure to treat four patients suffering from a life-threatening condition called pseudomembranous colitis, a condition caused by C. *difficile* infection and induced by antibiotic exposure. All four patients experienced a prompt recovery and were discharged from the hospital within days. Without this procedure, they likely would have died. Thereafter, more and more citations demonstrating the effectiveness of FMT in the treatment of C. *difficile* began to appear in the literature.

However, the very first description of FMT occurred much earlier than sixty years ago. In fact, references to the procedure date back 1,700 years and are found in Chinese literature written by Ge Hong, China's most famous alchemist. He wrote about the transmission of disease (especially fever-related disease) and was known for his teachings about food poisoning. In one of these ancient scrolls, he describes the administration of a human feces suspension by mouth for the treatment of severe diarrhea or food poisoning. This was in the fourth century! In the sixteenth century, also in China, Li Shinzen described administering a solution of fermented dried infant feces in a preparation called "yellow soup" for a variety of medical problems, including vomiting, constipation, fever, and diarrhea.[3] During World War II, German soldiers in Africa confirmed the efficacy of the Bedouin practice of consuming fresh warm camel feces as a treatment for bacterial dysentery.[4] Interestingly, in all the documentation we have dating back to 4th century China, there has never been a single, serious side effect reported from this procedure.[5]

So FMT isn't as novel as you might think. I recently had the opportunity to visit a team of researchers from Harvard and MIT who have created a nonprofit company called OpenBiome to make the procedure more widely available. They are harvesting fecal material from students at these institutions, processing them, and then shipping the specimens to more than 150 hospitals around America for use in treating C. *difficile.* Inspiration for this project came from the company's founders, who watched a loved one suffer through eighteen months of C. *difficile* and seven rounds of vancomycin before finally receiving a successful, life-changing FMT.

I may be among a small handful of clinicians in the world today encouraging this technique to treat brain disorders in select individuals, but that is going to change soon enough. I have no doubt that we'll see FMT increasingly used for other types of illnesses and disorders. New research is showing that FMT is very effective in treating Crohn's disease. And some physicians claim to have had great success using FMT to treat ulcerative colitis, celiac disease, chronic fatigue syndrome, and many brain-related disorders such as multiple sclerosis and Tourette syndrome. It's now being looked at for obesity, diabetes, and rheumatoid arthritis, as well as for Parkinson's disease and other neurological conditions. And it is my sincere hope that, based on the finding of elevated LPS in ALS, this devastating condition will soon be added to the list. In my own experience, I've even witnessed the power of FMT on children with autism, as you'll recall from the story of Jason.

One of the global pioneers today in recognizing the benefits of FMT is Dr. Thomas J. Borody. Born in Poland, he moved to Australia in 1960, where he received his medical degree and subsequently engaged in postgraduate research at the Mayo Clinic. Dr. Borody has been performing FMT for the past twenty-five years, first experimenting with its utility for C. *difficile* but then quickly moving on to other disorders that affect areas from the gut to the brain. Dr. Borody has fully embraced the science of gut bacteria's lead role in regulating inflammation and immunity. He has used FMT to successfully treat an array of diseases that involve the immune and neurological systems.[6, 7]

While Dr. Borody certainly has his critics, many others are now looking upon his work with respect, especially in light of the results he is getting. His published case reports are downright astonishing. In one, published in the *American Journal of Gastroenterology*, he revealed that alterations of the gut bacteria are seen in multiple sclerosis, Parkinson's disease, and myasthenia gravis, an autoimmune condition that often leads to severe weakness.[8] One of his most breathtaking cases is that of a thirty-year-old man with MS who received FMT for severe constipation. The patient also suffered from severe vertigo, difficulty with concentration, and leg weakness so bad that he needed to use a wheelchair. Moreover, he wasn't able to control his bladder, so he had a urinary catheter. Standard treatments, which included modulating his immune system with interferon, had failed this man. Taking another approach, Dr. Borody performed five FMT treatments. They led not only to resolution

of the constipation but also to progressive improvement of his MS symptoms. He regained the ability to walk and no longer needed the catheter.
Although he was deemed to be in remission, he remains well today—
fifteen years later.

The Commonwealth Scientific and Industrial Research Organisa-
tion (CSIRO) is Australia's national science agency and is one of the
largest and most diverse research agencies in the world. Their chief
research scientist, Dr. David Topping, was recently asked to comment on
Dr. Borody's work with FMT. He stated, "The interaction between microflora, particularly their products and their substrate, holds immense
potential for the management and prevention of serious diseases, colorectal cancer, inflammatory bowel disease, perhaps even conditions like
Alzheimer's, autism and Parkinson's."[9]

Now that you know how important your gut bacteria are in terms of
inflammation, immunity, and neurology, you can see that for me there
can be no going back. When you consider the fact that neurological disorders like autism, Alzheimer's, and Parkinson's currently have no cure
whatsoever, all of this latest science infuses me with hope. I love how Dr.
Robert Orenstein, of the Mayo Clinic in Arizona, puts it in an article
about FMT: "The microbiome of the gut is not inactive; it's diverse and
plays many roles in health and well-being that are just now being
explored. With molecular biology and the sequencing of these species,
this can only get bigger. It's like the beginning of the space program."[10]

EXCITING NEW TECHNOLOGIES

Another extraordinary example of cutting-edge medicine in development today is seen in the use of parasitic worm eggs to cure inflammatory
bowel disease (IBD).[11] Some 1.4 million people in the U.S. have IBD,
which is characterized by chronic or recurring adverse immune reaction
and inflammation of the gastrointestinal tract. Ulcerative colitis and

Crohn's disease are the two most common inflammatory bowel diseases. Clinical trials have just commenced in humans, but we already know a lot about how worms can lead to a cure through the work done on rhesus macaque monkeys, who can also suffer from their own version of IBD when in captivity. For a long time, veterinarians were at a loss as to how to treat these monkeys, who often suffered from dangerous weight loss and dehydration from the disease. But new research in just the last few years reveals that after giving the monkeys parasitic whipworm eggs, most of them recovered.[12]

To understand the changes that would occur in the monkeys' intestines, the researchers examined the lining of the monkeys' colons before and after treatment. Before treatment with the worm eggs, the monkeys had an abnormally high rate of one type of bacteria being attached to their colon linings, and this was presumably revving up the immune response unnecessarily and triggering IBD. This changed after treatment, as the bacterial communities shifted in their quantity and type. Such changes also had the effect of lowering inflammation by reducing the expression of certain genes in the monkeys' DNA.

To be sure, this particular study, done by a team at New York University Langone Medical Center and the University of California San Francisco, isn't the first of its kind. Small human trials have found that giving people the microscopic eggs of pig whipworm (or *Trichuris suis*) can diminish symptoms of IBD.[13] But for a long time scientists had no idea why the eggs were working. And now we can confidently explain the mechanism: Exposure to these eggs restores balance to the microbial communities that are sticking to the intestinal wall. (And no, the eggs don't "hatch" inside or pass through the stool.) I should add that IBD is rarely seen in underdeveloped countries where infection with parasitic worms in the gastrointestinal tract is commonplace. As with Alzheimer's disease, irritable bowel diseases are mainly seen in developed countries, such as the U.S. and European nations, a fact that again gives credibility to the hygiene hypothesis—that being too clean can backfire. Perhaps one day we may find more "parasite" therapies for IBD and other inflammatory diseases. Experimental work is already under way to see if worm eggs can treat colitis, asthma, rheumatoid arthritis, food allergies, and type 1 diabetes.

In the words of science writer Katherine Harmon Courage, "Perhaps just think of them as the caviar of probiotics."[14]

A BRAVE NEW WORLD

By the time you read this book, we will have mapped more organisms of the human microbiome than the number we currently — as I write — have on file, thanks to the Human Microbiome Project initiated by the National Institutes of Health in 2008. The NIH is supporting a coordinated effort to characterize our microbiome, with work being conducted at four sequencing centers: the J. Craig Venter Institute, Baylor College of Medicine, the Broad Institute, and Washington University School of Medicine. Certainly others will get involved, too, from both private and publically funded organizations. The project aims to identify the microbial communities in different parts of the body in thousands of individuals. This extensive sampling will help determine whether there is a core microbiome in each part and help scientists probe the relationship between health status and changes in the microbiome. At the University of Colorado, the American Gut Project is under way. Researchers there are testing about 7,000 stool samples sent in by donors, along with information about their diet, health, and lifestyle habits — a bonanza of data to mine.

But identifying the microbial populations that natively inhabit us will be just the beginning. We have to figure out what all that data means in terms of health or, conversely, disease. We also have to investigate the connections between the microbiome and lifestyle factors (such as how much alcohol we drink and how much sleep we get), as well as the elaborate interplay between the forces of genetics and microbial composition. And I can't wait to see what we discover. As I write this epilogue, the journal *Nature* has just published yet another article to sound the alarm. The headline says it all: "Gut-brain link grabs neuroscientists."[15] In it, the author writes that we're "only now starting to understand how gut bacteria may influence the brain" and that "[n]ow there is hard evidence linking conditions such as autism and depression to the gut's microbial residents."

Hard evidence indeed. The race to new cures for all of these maladies has begun. Welcome to a new era of medicine and personalized care.

Just over a decade ago I developed a close friendship with Dr. Amar Bose. If that name isn't familiar, you will no doubt recognize it when I explain that the sound system in your car was probably designed by his company. Dr. Bose built a career on exploring and transcending boundaries, not just in audio equipment but also in many areas of science and technology. I remember the day he proudly escorted me through his research laboratory, revealing projects that were building on incredibly futuristic product development ideas. We went from one laboratory to the next, and it was clear how proud he was of the work of his research scientists. But what was most memorable for me when I visited him that day was the 1911 quote by Belgian Nobel laureate Maurice Maeterlinck that was stenciled on the glass wall of Bose's private office. It really summed up the motivational force that led to Bose's great success: "At every crossway on the road that leads to the future, each progressive spirit is opposed by a thousand men assigned to guard the past."

Clearly there are those who will want to defend the past and even the status quo. That is to be expected. I believe it is far more important to break the bonds of these constraints and recognize that our most exciting and respected science is offering us an incredible opportunity to regain our health through the force wielded by the microbiome — the human brain maker. We can harness this inner power for our own betterment, as we are now at the crossway that leads to the future. Join the revolution.

Acknowledgments

A doctor writing a book for the lay public on a complex health topic needs extra-special help. I am deeply grateful to the following people who made this book possible:

My literary agent, Bonnie Solow, for your direction and ability to see the whole picture and keep things moving forward. I don't know what I enjoy more — working with you professionally or our dear friendship. You provided the initial spark years ago when we joined forces on *Grain Brain*. Thanks also for your steadfast attention to details, your acting as a supreme source of publishing advice, and your insightful stewardship. As before, you've gone beyond the call of duty.

Tracy Behar, my editor at Little, Brown, helped champion this work from the day it was a rough outline, knowing that this message could pave the way for a revolution in healthcare. Thank you for your editorial leadership and for helping me create a most succinct and practical book on such a complex topic. Thanks also to your incredible team, including Michael Pietsch, Reagan Arthur, Nicole Dewey, Heather Fain, Miriam Parker, Cathy Gruhn, Jonathan Jacobs, Ben Allen, Genevieve Nierman, and Kathryn Rogers.

Kristin Loberg, you have so totally captured my voice. Your unparalleled ability to transform my highly technical manuscript into text that can be embraced by so many will clearly facilitate a transformation in health.

Thank you Judith Choate, for graciously putting together the delicious recipes and spending more time in the kitchen making sure only the best dishes made the final cut.

To my indefatigable tech team at Digital Natives, for your work in steering my social media campaign.

To my dedicated staff at the Perlmutter Health Center. Your amazing support of my clinical work has made it possible for me to implement ideas that hopefully will become mainstream in years to come.

Thanks to James Murphy for your leadership role not only in this project, but in directing every aspect of our outreach. I so appreciate your ability to actualize the vision.

Joe Miller and Andrew Luer, thank you for your daily support as we move ahead toward what will clearly be an exciting future.

And finally, I wish to thank my wife, Leize, who has provided love and counsel throughout the creation of this work and all of our endeavors together over the last twenty-nine years.

Notes

The following is a partial list of scientific papers, books, articles, and online resources that you might find helpful in learning more about some of the ideas and concepts expressed in this book. This is by no means an exhaustive list, but it will get you started in taking a new perspective and living up to the principles of *Brain Maker*. Many of these citations relate with studies briefly mentioned or described in detail in the text. These materials can also open doors for further research and inquiry. If you do not see a reference listed here that was mentioned in the book, please visit the website, www.DrPerlmutter.com, where you can access more studies and an ongoing updated list of references.

Introduction: Bug Alert

1. C. Pritchard, A. Mayers, and D. Baldwin, "Changing Patterns of Neurological Mortality in the 10 Major Developed Countries—1979–2010," *Publ. Health* 127, no. 4 (April 2013): 357–68. See also Bournemouth University, "Brain Diseases Affecting More People and Starting Earlier Than Ever Before," *ScienceDaily*, May 10, 2013, accessed January 8, 2015, http://www.sciencedaily.com/releases/2013/05/130510075502.htm.
2. Michael D. Hurd *et al.*, "Monetary Costs of Dementia in the United States," *N. Engl. J. Med.* 368 (April 4, 2013): 1326–34.
3. "Statistics," NIMH RSS, accessed January 12, 2015, http://www.nimh.nih.gov/health/statistics/index.shtml.
4. Ibid.
5. "Depression," WHO, October 2012, accessed January 12, 2015, http://www.who.int/mediacentre/factsheets/fs369/en/.

6. Kate Torgovnick, "Why Do the Mentally Ill Die Younger?," *Time*, December 3, 2008, accessed January 15, 2015, http://content.time.com/time/health/article/0,8599,1863220,00.html.

7. "Headache Disorders," WHO, October 2012, accessed January 15, 2015, http://www.who.int/mediacentre/factsheets/fs277/en/.

8. "Do You Practice Headache Hygiene?," HOPE Health Letter, July 2014, https://www.hopehealth.com/reports/PDF/Headache-Hygiene.pdf.

9. "Frequently Asked Questions about Multiple Sclerosis," Multiple Sclerosis FAQs and MS Glossary, accessed January 12, 2015, http://www.mymsaa.org/about-ms/faq/.

10. "Multiple Sclerosis Statistics," Statistic Brain RSS, accessed January 12, 2015, http://www.statisticbrain.com/multiple-sclerosis-statistics/.

11. "Data & Statistics," Centers for Disease Control and Prevention, March 24, 2014, accessed January 12, 2015, http://www.cdc.gov/ncbddd/autism/data.html.

12. "NIH Human Microbiome Project Defines Normal Bacterial Makeup of the Body," U.S National Library of Medicine, accessed January 12, 2015, http://www.nih.gov/news/health/jun2012/nhgri-13.htm.

13. "Human Microbiome Project DACC—Home," Human Microbiome RSS, accessed January 12, 2015, http://hmpdacc.org/.

14. S. Reardon, "Gut-Brain Link Grabs Neuroscientists," *Nature* 515 (November 13, 2014): 175–77, doi: 10.1038/515175a.

15. This quote has long been attributed to Hippocrates, but in fact the phrase is not found in any of his writings. Although the link between dietary choices and health has been known and documented scientifically for centuries, even Hippocrates would agree that the concept of food should not be confused with the concept of medication. In 2013, Diana Cardenas of Paris Descartes University wrote a paper about this literary creation, in which she shows that at least one biomedical journal over the last thirty years has cited this mistaken phrase. But it still remains a good adage nonetheless, one that's relevant and true no matter who came up with it.

Chapter 1: Welcome Aboard

1. Dan Buettner, "The Island Where People Forget to Die," *New York Times Magazine*, October 24, 2012, http://www.nytimes.com/2012/10/28/magazine/the-island-where-people-forget-to-die.html.

2. D. B. Panagiotakos *et al.*, "Sociodemographic and Lifestyle Statistics of Oldest Old People (>80 Years) Living in Ikaria Island: The Ikaria Study," *Cardiol. Res. Pract.* 2011 (February 24, 2011): Article ID 679187, 7 pages.

3. "Link between Microbes and Obesity," MicrobeWiki, Kenyon College, accessed January 12, 2015, https://microbewiki.kenyon.edu/index.php/Link_Between_Microbes_and_Obesity.

4. "NIH Human Microbiome Project Defines Normal Bacterial Makeup of the Body," U.S National Library of Medicine, accessed January 12, 2015, http://www.nih.gov/news/health/jun2012/nhgri-13.htm.

5. "How Bacteria in the Gut Help Fight Off Viruses," NPR, accessed January 12, 2015, http://www.npr.org/blogs/goatsandsoda/2014/11/14/363375355/how-bacteria-in-the-gut-help-fight-off-viruses.

6. Adam Hadhazy, "Think Twice: How the Gut's 'Second Brain' Influences Mood and Well-Being," *Scientific American*, February 12, 2010, http://www.scientificamerican.com/article/gut-second-brain/.

7. Dr. Siri Carpenter, "That Gut Feeling," *Am. Psychol. Assoc.* 43, no. 8 (September 2012): 50, http://www.apa.org/monitor/2012/09/gut-feeling.aspx.

8. Ibid.

9. Ivana Semova *et al.*, "Microbiota Regulate Intestinal Absorption and Metabolism of Fatty Acids in the Zebrafish," *Cell Host & Microbe* 12, no. 3 (2012): 277. See also University of North Carolina School of Medicine, "Gut Microbes Help the Body Extract More Calories from Food," *ScienceDaily*, September 12, 2012, accessed January 8, 2015, http://www.sciencedaily.com/releases/2012/09/120912125114.htm.

10. N. Abdallah Ismail, "Frequency of Firmicutes and Bacteroidetes in Gut Microbiota in Obese and Normal Weight Egyptian Children and Adults," *Arch. Med. Sci.* 7, no. 3 (June 2011): 501–7, doi: 10.5114/aoms.2011.23418, Epub July 11, 2011.

11. H. Kumar *et al.*, "Gut Microbiota as an Epigenetic Regulator: Pilot Study Based on Whole-Genome Methylation Analysis. *mBio* 5, no. 6 (2014): e02113–14, doi:10.1128/mBio.02113-14.

12. "*Clostridium difficile* Infection," Centers for Disease Control and Prevention, March 1, 2013, accessed January 12, 2015, http://www.cdc.gov/HAI/organisms/cdiff/Cdiff_infect.html.

13. "For Medical Professionals: Quick, Inexpensive and a 90 Percent Cure Rate," accessed January 12, 2015, http://www.mayoclinic.org/medical-professionals/clinical-updates/digestive-diseases/quick-inexpensive-90-percent-cure-rate.

14. Tanya Lewis, "Go with Your Gut: How Bacteria May Affect Mental Health," *LiveScience*, October 8, 2013, accessed January 12, 2015, http://www.livescience.com/40255-how-bacteria-affect-mental-health.html.

15. K. Aagaard *et al.*, "The Placenta Harbors a Unique Microbiome," *Sci. Transl. Med.* 237, no. 6 (May 21, 2014): 237ra65.

16. Kerry Grens, "The Maternal Microbiome," *The Scientist*, May 21, 2014, http://www.the-scientist.com/?articles.view/articleNo/40038/title/The-Maternal-Microbiome/.

17. M. G. Dominguez-Bello *et al.*, "Delivery Mode Shapes the Acquisition and Structure of the Initial Microbiota across Multiple Body Habitats in Newborns," *Proc. Natl. Acad. Sci. USA* 107, no. 26 (June 29, 2010): 11971–75, Epub June 21, 2010.

18. M. B. Azad *et al.*, "Gut Microbiota of Healthy Canadian Infants: Profiles by Mode of Delivery and Infant Diet at 4 Months," *CMAJ* 185, no. 5 (March 19, 2013): 385–94, Epub February 11, 2013.

19. Canadian Medical Association Journal, "Infant Gut Microbiota Influenced by Cesarean Section and Breastfeeding Practices; May Impact Long-Term Health," *ScienceDaily*, February 11, 2013, accessed January 8, 2015, http://www.sciencedaily .com/releases/2013/02/130211134842.htm.

20. Martin J. Blasser, *Missing Microbes* (New York: Henry Holt, 2014).

21. Ibid, 99.

22. H. Makino *et al.*, "Mother-to-Infant Transmission of Intestinal Bifidobacterial Strains Has an Impact on the Early Development of Vaginally Delivered Infant's Microbiota," *PLoS One* 11, no. 8 (November 14, 2013): e78331.

23. Sarah Glynn, "C-Section Babies 5 Times More Likely to Develop Allergies," *Medical News Today*, February 27, 2013, accessed January 12, 2015, http://www.medical newstoday.com/articles/256915.php.

24. Shahrokh Amiri *et al.*, "Pregnancy-Related Maternal Risk Factors of Attention-Deficit Hyperactivity Disorder: A Case-Control Study," *ISRN Pediat.* 2012 (2012), http://dx.doi.org/10.5402/2012/458064.

25. E. J. Glasson, "Perinatal Factors and the Development of Autism: A Population Study," *Arch. Gen. Psychiatry* 61, no. 6 (June 2004): 618–27.

26. E. Decker *et al.*, "Cesarean Delivery Is Associated with Celiac Disease but Not Inflammatory Bowel Disease in Children," *Pediatrics* 125, no. 6 (June 2010), http://pediatrics.aappublications.org/content/early/2010/05/17/peds.2009-2260 .full.pdf.

27. H. A. Goldani *et al.*, "Cesarean Delivery Is Associated with an Increased Risk of Obesity in Adulthood in a Brazilian Birth Cohort Study," *Am. J. Clin. Nutr.* 93, no. 6 (June 2011): 1344–47, doi: 10.3945/ajcn.110.010033, Epub April 20, 2011.

28. C. C. Patterson *et al.*, "A Case-Control Investigation of Perinatal Risk Factors for Childhood IDDM in Northern Ireland and Scotland," *Diabetes Care* 17, no. 5 (May 1994): 376–81.

29. Karen Kaplan, "Diabetes Increases the Risk of Dementia and Alzheimer's Disease," *Los Angeles Times*, September 20, 2011, accessed January 12, 2015, http://articles .latimes.com/2011/sep/20/news/la-heb-diabetes-dementia-alzheimers-20110920.

30. Nell Lake, "Labor, Interrupted," *Harvard Magazine*, November–December 2012, accessed January 12, 2015, http://harvardmagazine.com/2012/11/labor-interrupted. See also "Births—Method of Delivery," Centers for Disease Control and Prevention, February 25, 2014, accessed January 12, 2015, http://www.cdc.gov/nchs/fastats/ delivery.htm.

31. W. P. Witt *et al.*, "Determinants of Cesarean Delivery in the US: A Lifecourse Approach," *Matern. Child Health J.* 1, no. 19 (January 2015): 84–93.

32. L. J. Funkhouser and S. R. Bordenstein, "Mom Knows Best: The Universality of Maternal Microbial Transmission," *PLoS Biol.* 11, no. 8 (2013), doi: 10.1371/journal .pbio.1001631, Epub August 20, 2013.

33. Erica Sonnenburg and Justin Sonnenburg, "Starving Our Microbial Self: The Deleterious Consequences of a Diet Deficient in Microbiota-Accessible Carbohydrates," *Cell Metab.* 20, no. 5 (November 4, 2014): 779–86.

34. Emily Eakin, "The Excrement Experiment," *New Yorker*, December 1, 2014.

35. Semova *et al.*, "Microbiota Regulate Intestinal Absorption and Metabolism of Fatty Acids." See also K. Brown *et al.*, "Diet-Induced Dysbiosis of the Intestinal Microbiota and the Effects on Immunity and Disease," *Nutrients* 8, no. 4 (August 2012): 1095–1119, Epub August 21, 2012.

36. M. Fox *et al.*, "Hygiene and the World Distribution of Alzheimer's Disease," *Evol. Med. Publ. Health*, 2013, doi: 10.1093/emph/eot015. See also University of Cambridge, "Better Hygiene in Wealthy Nations May Increase Alzheimer's Risk, Study Suggests," *ScienceDaily*, accessed January 8, 2015, http://www.sciencedaily.com/ releases/2013/09/130904105347.htm. The images on page 41 were created based on the images and data featured in the original study by Fox and colleagues.

37. "Who's in Control: The Human Host or the Microbiome?," Organic Fitness, September 27, 2014, accessed January 12, 2015, http://organicfitness.com/whos-in -control-the-human-host-or-the-microbiome/.

Chapter 2: Belly and Brain on Fire

1. David Perlmutter, "Why We Can and Must Focus on Preventing Alzheimer's," *Daily Beast*, August 22, 2013, accessed January 12, 2015, http://www.thedailybeast .com/articles/2013/08/22/why-we-can-and-must-focus-on-preventing-alzheimer-s .html.

2. Gina Kolata, "An Unusual Partnership to Tackle Stubborn Diseases," *New York Times*, February 5, 2014, A14.

3. R. S. Doody *et al.*, "Phase 3 Trials of Solanezumab for Mild-to-Moderate Alzheimer's Disease," *N. Engl. J. Med.* 370, no. 4 (January 23, 2014): 311–21, doi: 10.1056/ NEJMoa1312889.

4. S. Salloway *et al.*, "Two Phase 3 Trials of Bapineuzumab in Mild-to-Moderate Alzheimer's Disease," *N. Engl. J. Med.* 370, no. 4 (January 23, 2014): 322–33, doi: 10.1056/NEJMoa1304839.

5. L. S. Schneider *et al.*, "Lack of Evidence for the Efficacy of Memantine in Mild Alzheimer Disease," *Arch. Neurol.* 68, no. 8 (August 2011): 991–98, doi: 10.1001/ archneurol.2011.69, Epub April 11, 2011.

6. Alzheimer's Association, *2012 Alzheimer's Disease Facts and Figures*, http://www.alz .org/downloads/facts_figures_2012.pdf.

7. P. Crane *et al.*, "Glucose Levels and Risk of Dementia," *N. Engl. J. Med.* 2013, no. 369 (August 8, 2013): 540–48, doi: 10.1056/NEJMoa1215740.

8. E. H. Martinez-Lapiscina *et al.*, "Mediterranean Diet Improves Cognition: The PREDIMED-NAVARRA Randomised Trial," *J. Neurol. Neurosurg. Psychiatry* 84, no. 12 (December 2013): 1318–25, doi: 10.1136/jnnp-2012-304792, Epub May 13, 2013. Also see E. H. Martinez-Lapiscina *et al.*, "Virgin Olive Oil Supplementation and Long-term Cognition: The PREDIMED-NAVARRA Randomized Trial," *J. Nutr. Health Aging* 17, no. 6 (2013): 544–52.

9. "Alzheimer's Disease and Inflammation," Overview Alzheimer's Disease and Inflammation Lab: Pritam Das, accessed January 12, 2015, http://www.mayo.edu/research/labs/alzheimers-disease-inflammation/overview.

10. H. Fillit *et al.*, "Elevated Circulating Tumor Necrosis Factor Levels in Alzheimer's Disease," *Neurosci. Lett.* 129, no. 2 (August 19, 1991): 318–20. The image on page 48 is based on data from the following study: H. Bruunsgaard, "The Clinical Impact of Systemic Low-Level Inflammation in Elderly Populations. With Special Reference to Cardiovascular Disease, Dementia and Mortality," *Dan. Med. Bull.* 53, no. 3 (August 2006): 285–309.

11. A. J. Gearing *et al.*, "Processing of Tumour Necrosis Factor-Alpha Precursor by Metalloproteinases," *Nature* 370, no. 6490 (August 1994): 555–57.

12. B. B. Aggarwal, S. C. Gupta, and J. H. Kim, "Historical Perspectives on Tumor Necrosis Factor and Its Superfamily: 25 Years Later, a Golden Journey," *Blood* 119, no. 3 (January 19, 2012): 651–65.

13. M. Sastre *et al.*, "Contribution of Inflammatory Processes to Alzheimer's Disease: Molecular Mechanisms," *Int. J. Dev. Neurosci.* 24, no. 2–3 (April–May 2006): 167–76, Epub February 10, 2006.

14. Suzanne M. de la Monte and Jack R. Wands, "Alzheimer's Disease Is Type 3 Diabetes—Evidence Reviewed," *J. Diabetes Sci. Technol.* 2, no. 6 (November 2008): 1101–13. Published online November 2008.

15. J. Qin *et al.*, "A Metagenome-wide Association Study of Gut Microbiota in Type 2 Diabetes," *Nature* 490, no. 7418 (October 4, 2012): 55–60. doi: 10.1038/nature11450. Epub September 26, 2012. Also see Frank Ervolino, "Could Gut Flora Be Linked to Diabetes?," Vitamin Research Products, accessed January 12, 2015, http://www.vrp.com/digestive-health/digestive-health/could-gut-flora-be-linked-to-diabetes.

16. Yong Zhang and Heping Zhang, "Microbiota Associated with Type 2 Diabetes and Its Related Complications," *Food Sci. Human Wellness* 2, nos. 3–4 (September–December 2013): 167–72, http://www.sciencedirect.com/science/article/pii/S2213453013000451.

17. J. M. Hill *et al.*, "The Gastrointestinal Tract Microbiome and Potential Link to Alzheimer's Disease," *Front. Neurol.* 5 (April 4, 2014): 43, doi: 10.3389/fneur.2014.00043, eCollection 2014.

18. G. Weinstein *et al.*, "Serum Brain-Derived Neurotrophic Factor and the Risk for Dementia: The Framingham Heart Study," *JAMA Neurol.* 71, no. 1 (January 2014): 55–61, doi: 10.1001/jamaneurol.2013.4781.

19. Ibid.

20. American Society for Microbiology, "Intestinal Bacteria Produce Neurotransmitter, Could Play Role in Inflammation," *ScienceDaily*, accessed January 12, 2015, http://www.sciencedaily.com/releases/2012/06/120617142536.htm.

21. J. R. Turner, "Intestinal Mucosal Barrier Function in Health and Disease," *Nat. Rev. Immunol.* 9, no. 11 (November 2009): 799–809, doi: 10.1038/nri2653.

22. A. Fasano, "Zonulin and Its Regulation of Intestinal Barrier Function: The Biological Door to Inflammation, Autoimmunity, and Cancer," *Physiol. Rev.* 91, no. 1 (January 2011): 151–75, doi: 10.1152/physrev.00003.2008.

23. M. M. Welling, R. J. Nabuurs, and L. van der Weerd, "Potential Role of Antimicrobial Peptides in the Early Onset of Alzheimer's Disease," *Alzheimers Dement.* 11, no. 1 (January 2015): 51–7. doi: 10.1016/j.jalz.2013.12.020. Epub 2014 Mar 15.

24. J. R. Jackson *et al.*, "Neurologic and Psychiatric Manifestations of Celiac Disease and Gluten Sensitivity," *Psychiatr. Q.* 83, no. 1 (March 2012): 91–102, doi: 10.1007/s11126-011-9186-y.

25. Marielle Suzanne Kahn, "A Potential Role for LPS-Induced Inflammation in the Induction of Alzheimer's Disease-Related Pathology and Cognitive Deficits," Master's thesis, Texas Christian University, Pub number: 1491006, http://gradworks.umi.com/14/91/1491006.html.

26. M. Kahn *et al.*, "A Potential Role for LPS-Induced Inflammation in the Induction of Alzheimer's Disease-Related Pathology and Cognitive Deficits," Texas Christian University, http://www.srs.tcu.edu/previous_posters/Interdisciplinary/2011/122-Kahn-Chumley.pdf.

27. J. W. Lee *et al.*, "Neuro-inflammation Induced by Lipopolysaccharide Causes Cognitive Impairment through Enhancement of Beta-Amyloid Generation," *J. Neuroinflamm.* 5 (August 29, 2008): 37, doi: 10.1186/1742-2094-5-37.

28. Z. Guan and J. Fang, "Peripheral Immune Activation by Lipopolysaccharide Decreases Neurotrophins in the Cortex and Hippocampus in Rats," *Brain Behav. Immun.* 20, no. 1 (January 2006): 64–71.

29. R. Zhang *et al.*, "Circulating Endotoxin and Systemic Immune Activation in Sporadic Amyotrophic Lateral Sclerosis (sALS)," *J. Neuroimmunol.* 206, no. 1–2 (January 3, 2009): 121–24, doi: 10.1016/j.jneuroim.2008.09.017, Epub November 14, 2008. The images on page 58 are based on data from this study.

30. Ibid.

31. C. B. Forsyth *et al.*, "Increased Intestinal Permeability Correlates with Sigmoid Mucosa Alpha-Synuclein Staining and Endotoxin Exposure Markers in Early Parkinson's Disease," *PLoS One* 6, no. 12 (2011): e28032, doi: 10.1371/journal.pone.0028032, Epub 2011 December 1, 2011.

32. "Manifestations of Low Vitamin B12 Levels," Centers for Disease Control and Prevention, June 29, 2009, accessed January 12, 2015, http://www.cdc.gov/ncbddd/b12/manifestations.html.

33. H. W. Baik and R. M. Russell, "Vitamin B12 Deficiency in the Elderly," *Ann. Rev. Nutr.* 19 (1999): 357–77.

34. P. M. Kris-Etherton *et al.*, "Polyunsaturated Fatty Acids in the Food Chain in the United States," *Am. J. Clin. Nutr.* 71, Suppl. 1 (January 2000): 179S–88S.

35. M. H. Eskelinen *et al.*, "Midlife Coffee and Tea Drinking and the Risk of Late-Life Dementia: A Population-Based CAIDE Study," *J. Alzheimers Dis.* 16, no. 1 (2009): 85–91, doi: 10.3233/JAD-2009-0920.

36. Ibid.

37. Janet Raloff, "A Gut Feeling about Coffee," *ScienceNews*, July 26, 2007, https://www.sciencenews.org/blog/food-thought/gut-feeling-about-coffee.

38. M. Jaquet *et al.*, "Impact of Coffee Consumption on the Gut Microbiota: A Human Volunteer Study," *J. Food Microbiol.* 130, no. 2 (March 31, 2009): 117–21, doi: 10.1016/j.ijfoodmicro.2009.01.011, Epub January 23, 2009.

39. T. E. Cowan *et al.*, "Chronic Coffee Consumption in the Diet-Induced Obese Rat: Impact on Gut Microbiota and Serum Metabolomics," *J. Nutr. Biochem.* 25, no. 4 (April 2014): 489–95, doi: 10.1016/j.jnutbio.2013.12.009, Epub January 30, 2014.

40. David Perlmutter and Alberto Villoldo, *Power of Your Brain* (New York: Hay House, 2011).

41. Nick Lane, *Power, Sex, and Suicide: Mitochondria and the Meaning of Life* (New York: Oxford University Press, 2006); page 207.

42. C. O'Gorman *et al.*, "Environmental Risk Factors for Multiple Sclerosis: A Review with a Focus on Molecular Mechanisms," *Int. J. Mol. Sci.* 13, no. 9 (2012): 11718–52, doi: 10.3390/ijms130911718, Epub September 18, 2012.

43. S. Conradi *et al.*, "Breastfeeding Is Associated with Lower Risk for Multiple Sclerosis," *Mult. Scler.* 19, no. 5 (April 2013): 553–58, doi: 10.1177/1352458512459683, Epub September 4, 2012.

Chapter 3: Is Your Belly Depressed?

1. Roni Caryn Rabin, "A Glut of Antidepressants," *New York Times*, August 12, 2013, http://well.blogs.nytimes.com/2013/08/12/a-glut-of-antidepressants/.

2. "Astounding Increase in Antidepressant Use by Americans—Harvard Health Blog," *Harvard Health Blog* RSS, October 20, 2011, accessed January 12, 2015, http://www.health.harvard.edu/blog/astounding-increase-in-antidepressant-use-by-americans-201110203624.

3. "Countries of the World: Gross National Product (GNP) Distribution—2005," accessed January 12, 2015, http://www.studentsoftheworld.info/infopays/rank/PNB2.html.

4. Kathryn Roethel, "Antidepressants—Nation's Top Prescription," *SFGate*, November 13, 2012, accessed January 12, 2015, http://www.sfgate.com/health/article/Antidepressants-nation-s-top-prescription-4034392.php.

5. "REPORT: Turning Attention to ADHD," accessed January 12, 2015, http://lab.express-scripts.com/insights/industry-updates/report-turning-attention-to-adhd.

6. "Depression (Major Depressive Disorder): Selective Serotonin Reuptake Inhibitors (SSRIs)," accessed January 12, 2015, http://www.mayoclinic.org/diseases-conditions/depression/in-depth/ssris/art-20044825.

7. L. Desbonnet *et al.*, "The Probiotic *Bifidobacteria infantis*: An Assessment of Potential Antidepressant Properties in the Rat," *J. Psychiatr. Res.* 43, no. 2 (December 2008): 164–74, doi: 10.1016/j.jpsychires.2008.03.009, Epub May 5, 2008.

8. A. C. Bested *et al.*, "Intestinal Microbiota, Probiotics and Mental Health: From Metchnikoff to Modern Advances: Part II—Contemporary Contextual Research," *Gut Pathog.* 5, no. 1 (March 2013): 3, doi: 10.1186/1757-4749-5-3. See also A. C. Bested *et al.*, "Intestinal Microbiota, Probiotics and Mental Health: From Metchnikoff to Modern Advances: Part III—Convergence toward Clinical Trials," *Gut Pathog.* 5, no. 1 (March 16, 2013): 4, doi: 10.1186/1757-4749-5-4.

9. A. Ferrao and J. E. Kilman, "Experimental Toxic Approach to Mental Illness," *Psychiatr. Q.* 7 (1933): 115–53.

10. G. M. Khandaker *et al.*, "Association of Serum Interleukin 6 and C-Reactive Protein in Childhood with Depression and Psychosis in Young Adult Life: A Population-Based Longitudinal Study," *JAMA Psychiatry* 71, no. 10 (October 2014): 1121–28, doi: 10.1001/jamapsychiatry.2014.1332.

11. Maria Almond, "Depression and Inflammation: Examining the Link," *Curr. Psychiatry* 6, no. 12 (2013): 24–32.

12. E. Painsipp *et al.*, "Prolonged Depression-like Behavior Caused by Immune Challenge: Influence of Mouse Strain and Social Environment," *PLoS One* 6, no. 6 (2011): e20719, doi: 10.1371/journal.pone.0020719, Epub June 6, 2011.

13. M. Udina *et al.*, "Interferon-Induced Depression in Chronic Hepatitis C: A Systematic Review and Meta-analysis," *J. Clin. Psychiatry* 73, no. 8 (August 2012): 1128–38, doi: 10.4088/JCP.12r07694.

14. N. Vogelzangs *et al.*, "Association of Depressive Disorders, Depression Characteristics and Antidepressant Medication with Inflammation," *Transl. Psychiatry* 2 (February 21, 2012): e79, doi: 10.1038/tp.2012.8.

15. E. Lopez-Garcia *et al.*, "Major Dietary Patterns Are Related to Plasma Concentrations of Markers of Inflammation and Endothelial Dysfunction," *Am. J. Clin. Nutr.* 80, no. 4 (October 2004): 1029–35.

16. S. Liu *et al.*, "Relation between a Diet with a High Glycemic Load and Plasma Concentrations of High-Sensitivity C-Reactive Protein in Middle-Aged Women," *Am. J. Clin. Nutr.* 75, no. 3 (March 2002): 492–98.

17. "Diabetes: What's the Connection between Diabetes and Depression: How Can I Cope If I Have Both?," Mayo Clinic, accessed January 12, 2015, http://www.mayo clinic.org/diseases-conditions/diabetes/expert-answers/diabetes-and-depression/faq-20057904.

18. A. Pan et al., "Bidirectional Association between Depression and Type 2 Diabetes Mellitus in Women," *Arch. Intern. Med.* 170, no. 21 (November 22, 2010): 1884–91, doi: 10.1001/archinternmed.2010.356.

19. F. S. Luppino et al., "Overweight, Obesity, and Depression: A Systematic Review and Meta-analysis of Longitudinal Studies," *JAMA Psychiatry* 67, no. 3 (March 2010): 220–9.

20. M. Maes et al., "The Gut-Brain Barrier in Major Depression: Intestinal Mucosal Dysfunction with an Increased Translocation of LPS from Gram Negative Entero-bacteria (Leaky Gut) Plays a Role in the Inflammatory Pathophysiology of Depression," *Neuro. Endocrinol. Lett.* 29, no. 1 (February 2008): 117–24. The image on page 78 is based on data from this study.

21. Ibid.

22. Bested et al., "Intestinal Microbiota," Part II.

23. A. Sanchez-Villegas et al., "Association of the Mediterranean Dietary Pattern with the Incidence of Depression: The Seguimiento Universidad de Navarra/University of Navarra Follow-Up (SUN) Cohort," *Arch. Gen. Psychiatry* 66, no. 10 (October 2009): 1090–98, doi: 10.1001/archgenpsychiatry.2009.129.

24. Bested et al., "Intestinal Microbiota," Part II.

25. M. E. Benros et al., "Autoimmune Diseases and Severe Infections as Risk Factors for Mood Disorders: A Nationwide Study," *JAMA Psychiatry* 70, no. 8 (August 2013): 812–20, doi: 10.1001/jamapsychiatry.2013.1111.

26. Sonia Shoukat and Thomas W. Hale, "Breastfeeding in Infancy May Reduce the Risk of Major Depression in Adulthood," Texas Tech University Health Sciences Center, September 18, 2012, http://www.infantrisk.com/content/breastfeeding-infancy-may-reduce-risk-major-depression-adulthood-1.

27. K. M. Neufeld et al., "Reduced Anxiety-like Behavior and Central Neurochemical Change in Germ-Free Mice," *Neurogastroenterol. Motil.* 23, no. 3 (March 2011): 255–64, e119, doi: 10.1111/j.1365-2982.2010.01620.x, Epub November 5, 2010.

28. P. Bercik et al., "The Intestinal Microbiota Affect Central Levels of Brain-Derived Neurotropic Factor and Behavior in Mice," *Gastroenterology* 141, no. 2 (August 2011): 599–609, 609.e1–3, doi: 10.1053/j.gastro.2011.04.052, Epub April 30, 2011.

29. Carrie Arnold, "Gut Feelings: The Future of Psychiatry May Be Inside Your Stomach," *The Verge*, August 21, 2013, http://www.theverge.com/2013/8/21/4595712/gut-feelings-the-future-of-psychiatry-may-be-inside-your-stomach.

30. K. Tillisch et al., "Consumption of Fermented Milk Product with Probiotic Modulates Brain Activity," *Gastroenterology* 144, no. 7 (June 2013): 1394–401,

1401.e1–4, doi: 10.1053/j.gastro.2013.02.043, Epub March 6, 2013. Also see E. A. Mayer *et al.*, "Gut Microbes and the Brain: Paradigm Shift in Neuroscience," *J. Neurosci.* 34, no. 46 (November 12, 2014): 15490–96, doi: 10.1523/JNEUROSCI .3299-14.2014.

31. Rachel Champeau, "Changing Gut Bacteria through Diet Affects Brain Function, UCLA Study Shows," UCLA Newsroom, May 28, 2013, http://newsroom.ucla.edu/ releases/changing-gut-bacteria-through-245617.

32. J. A. Foster and K. A. McVey, "Gut-Brain Axis: How the Microbiome Influences Anxiety and Depression," *Trends Neurosci.* 36, no. 5 (May 2013): 305–12, doi: 10.1016/j.tins.2013.01.005, Epub February 4, 2013.

33. T. Vanuytsel *et al.*, "Psychological Stress and Corticotropin-Releasing Hormone Increase Intestinal Permeability in Humans by a Mast Cell-Dependent Mechanism," *Gut* 63, no. 8 (August 2014): 1293–99, doi: 10.1136/gutjnl-2013-305690, Epub October 23, 2013.

34. N. Sudo *et al.*, "Postnatal Microbial Colonization Programs the Hypothalamic-Pituitary-Adrenal System for Stress Response in Mice," *J. Physiol.* 558, pt. 1 (July 2004): 263–75. Epub May 7, 2004.

35. J. M. Kreuger and J. A. Majde, "Microbial Products and Cytokines in Sleep and Fever Regulation," *Crit. Rev. Immunol.* 14, no 3–4 (1994): 355–79.

36. J. Glaus *et al.*, "Associations between Mood, Anxiety or Substance Use Disorders and Inflammatory Markers after Adjustment for Multiple Covariates in a Population-Based Study," *J. Psychiatr. Res.* 58 (November 2014): 36–45, doi: 10.1016/j.jpsychires .2014.07.012, Epub July 22, 2014.

37. A. E. Autry and L. M. Monteggia, "Brain-Derived Neurotrophic Factor and Neuro-psychiatric Disorders," *Pharmacol. Rev.* 64, no. 2 (April 2012): 238–58, doi: 10.1124/ pr.111.005108, Epub March 8, 2012.

38. J. Coplan *et al.*, "Persistent Elevations of Cerebrospinal Fluid Concentrations of Corticotropin-Releasing Factor in Adult Nonhuman Primates Exposed to Early-Life Stressors: Implications for the Pathophysiology of Mood and Anxiety Disorders," *Proc. Natl. Acad. Sci. USA* 93 (February 1996): 1619–23, http://www.ncbi .nlm.nih.gov/pmc/articles/PMC39991/pdf/pnas01508-0266.pdf.

39. Bested *et al.*, "Intestinal Microbiota," Part II.

40. "Anxiety Disorders," NIMH RSS, accessed January 12, 2015, http://www.nimh.nih .gov/health/publications/anxiety-disorders/index.shtml?rf=53414.

41. J. A. Bravo *et al.*, "Ingestion of *Lactobacillus* Strain Regulates Emotional Behavior and Central GABA Receptor Expression in a Mouse via the Vagus Nerve," *Proc. Natl. Acad. Sci. USA* 108, no. 38 (September 20, 2011): 16050–55, doi: 10.1073/ pnas.1102999108, Epub August 29, 2011.

42. University College Cork, "Mind-Altering Microbes: Probiotic Bacteria May Lessen Anxiety and Depression." *ScienceDaily*, accessed January 12, 2015, http://www .sciencedaily.com/releases/2011/08/110829164601.htm.

43. K. Schmidt *et al.*, "Prebiotic Intake Reduces the Waking Cortisol Response and Alters Emotional Bias in Healthy Volunteers," *Psychopharmacology* (Berl.) (December 3, 2014) [Epub ahead of print].

44. Bested *et al.*, "Intestinal Microbiota," Part II.

45. Barry Sears, "ADHD: An Inflammatory Condition," *Psychology Today*, July 20, 2011, http://www.psychologytoday.com/blog/in-the-zone/201107/adhd-inflammatory -condition.

46. Alan Schwarz, "Thousands of Toddlers Are Medicated for A.D.H.D., Report Finds, Raising Worries," *New York Times*, May 16, 2014, accessed January 12, 2015, http:// www.nytimes.com/2014/05/17/us/among-experts-scrutiny-of-attention-disorder -diagnoses-in-2-and-3-year-olds.html.

47. KJ Dell'Antonia, "The New Inequality for Toddlers: Less Income; More Ritalin," *New York Times*, Motherlode, May 16, 2014, http://parenting.blogs.nytimes.com/ 2014/05/16/the-new-inequality-for-toddlers-less-income-more-ritalin/.

48. T. Lempo *et al.*, "Altered Gene Expression in the Prefrontal Cortex of Young Rats Induced by the ADHD Drug Atomoxetine," *Prog. Neuropsychopharmacol. Biol. Psychiatry* 40 (January 10, 2013): 221–28, doi: 10.1016/j.pnpbp.2012.08.012, Epub August 30, 2012.

49. J. R. Burgess *et al.*, "Long-Chain Polyunsaturated Fatty Acids in Children with Attention-Deficit Hyperactivity Disorder," *Am. J. Clin. Nutr.* 71, Suppl. 1 (January 2000): 327S–30S.

50. Ibid.

51. E. A. Curran *et al.*, "Research Review: Birth by Caesarean Section and Development of Autism Spectrum Disorder and Attention-Deficit/Hyperactivity Disorder: A Systematic Review and Meta-analysis," *J. Child Psychol. Psychiatry* (October 27, 2014), doi: 10.1111/jcpp.12351 [Epub ahead of print].

52. C. McKeown *et al.*, "Association of Constipation and Fecal Incontinence with Attention-Deficit/Hyperactivity Disorder," *Pediatrics* 132, no. 5 (November 2013): e1210–15, doi: 10.1542/peds.2013-1580, Epub October 21, 2013.

53. H. Niederhofer, "Association of Attention-Deficit/Hyperactivity Disorder and Celiac Disease: A Brief Report," *Prim. Care Companion CNS Disord.* 13, no. 3 (2011), doi: 10.4088/PCC.10br01104.

54. L. M. Pelsser *et al.*, "Effects of a Restricted Elimination Diet on the Behaviour of Children with Attention-Deficit Hyperactivity Disorder (INCA Study): A Randomised Controlled Trial," *Lancet* 377, no. 9764 (February 5, 2011): 494–503, doi: 10.1016/S0140-6736(10)62227-1.

55. R. A. Edden *et al.*, "Reduced GABA Concentration in Attention-Deficit/Hyperactivity Disorder," *Arch. Gen. Psychiatry* 69, no. 7 (July 2012): 750–53, doi: 10.1001/ archgenpsychiatry.2011.2280.

56. E. Barrett *et al.*, "γ-Aminobutyric Acid Production by Culturable Bacteria from the Human Intestine," *J. Appl. Microbiol.* 113, no. 2 (August 2012): 411–17, doi: 10.1111/ j.1365-2672.2012.05344.x, Epub June 15, 2012.

57. J. Luo *et al.*, "Ingestion of Lactobacillus Strain Reduces Anxiety and Improves Cognitive Function in the Hyperammonemia Rat," *Sci. China Life Sci.* 57, no. 3 (March 2014): 327–35, doi: 10.1007/s11427-014-4615-4, Epub February 19, 2014.

58. M. Messaoudi *et al.*, "Assessment of Psychotropic-like Properties of a Probiotic Formulation (*Lactobacillus helveticus* R0052 and *Bifidobacterium longum* R0175) in Rats and Human Subjects," *Br. J. Nutr.* 105, no. 5 (March 2011): 755–64, doi: 10.1017/S0007114510004319, Epub October 26, 2010.

59. "Impulsive versus Controlled Men: Disinhibited Brains and Disinhibited Behavior," Press Release, Elsevier, November 3, 2011, http://www.elsevier.com/about/press-releases/research-and-journals/impulsive-versus-controlled-men-disinhibited-brains-and-disinhibited-behavior. See also D. J. Hayes *et al.*, "Brain γ-Aminobutyric Acid: A Neglected Role in Impulsivity," *Eur. J. Neurosci.* 39, no. 11 (June 2014): 1921–32, doi: 10.1111/ejn.12485, Epub January 27, 2014.

60. A. Draper *et al.*, "Increased GABA Contributes to Enhanced Control over Motor Excitability in Tourette Syndrome," *Curr. Biol.* 24, no. 19 (October 6, 2014): 2343–47, doi: 10.1016/j.cub.2014.08.038, Epub September 25, 2014. See also A. Lerner *et al.*, "Widespread Abnormality of the γ-Aminobutyric Acid-Ergic System in Tourette Syndrome," *Brain* 135, pt. 6 (June 2012): 1926–36, doi: 10.1093/brain/aws104, Epub May 10, 2012.

61. K. L. Harding *et al.*, "Outcome-Based Comparison of Ritalin versus Food-Supplement Treated Children with AD/HD," *Altern. Med. Rev.* 8, no. 3 (August 2003): 319–30, http://alternativementalhealth.com/articles/gant.pdf.

62. P. M. Kidd, "Attention Deficit/Hyperactivity Disorder (ADHD) in Children: Rationale for Its Integrative Management," *Altern. Med. Rev.* 5, no. 5 (October 2000): 402–28.

63. L. J. Stevens *et al.*, "Dietary Sensitivities and ADHD Symptoms: Thirty-Five Years of Research," *Clin. Pediatr.* (Phila.) 50, no. 4 (April 2011): 279–93, doi: 10.1177/0009922810384728, Epub December 2, 2010.

Chapter 4: How Your Intestinal Flora Can Make You Fat and Brainsick

1. "Obesity," WHO, accessed January 12, 2015, http://www.who.int/topics/obesity/en/.

2. "An Epidemic of Obesity: U.S. Obesity Trends," The Nutrition Source, accessed January 12, 2015, http://www.hsph.harvard.edu/nutritionsource/an-epidemic-of-obesity/.

3. "Obesity and Overweight," WHO, accessed January 12, 2015, http://www.who.int/mediacentre/factsheets/fs311/en/.

4. Meryl C. Vogt *et al.*, "Neonatal Insulin Action Impairs Hypothalamic Neurocircuit Formation in Response to Maternal High-Fat Feeding" *Cell* 156, no. 3 (January, 2014): 495–509, doi: http://dx.doi.org/10.1016/j.cell.2014.01.008.

5. N. Ashley *et al.*, "Maternal High-fat Diet and Obesity Compromise Fetal Hematopoiesis," Molecular Metabolism 2014; DOI: 10.1016/j.molmet.2014.11.001

6. C. De Filippo *et al.*, "Impact of Diet in Shaping Gut Microbiota Revealed by a Comparative Study in Children from Europe and Rural Africa," *Proc. Natl. Acad. Sci. USA* 107, no. 33 (August 17, 2010): 14691–96, doi: 10.1073/pnas.1005963107, Epub August 2, 2010. The images on pages 99 and 100 reflect data from this study.

7. Ibid. Also see Helen Pearson, "Fat People Harbor 'Fat' Microbes," *Nature*, December 20, 2006, http://www.nature.com/news/2006/061218/full/news061218-6.html.

8. M. A. O'Malley and K. Stotz, "Intervention, Integration and Translation in Obesity Research: Genetic, Developmental and Metaorganismal Approaches," *Philos. Ethics Humanit. Med.* 6 (January 2011): 2, doi: 10.1186/1747-5341-6-2.

9. H. D. Holscher *et al.*, "Fiber Supplementation Influences Phylogenetic Structure and Functional Capacity of the Human Intestinal Microbiome: Follow-Up of a Randomized Controlled Trial," *Am. J. Clin. Nutr.* 101, no. 1 (January 2015): 55–64, doi: 10.3945/ajcn.114.092064, Epub November 12, 2014.

10. De Filippo *et al.*, "Impact of Diet in Shaping Gut Microbiota." See also H. Tilg and A. Kaser, "Gut Microbiome, Obesity, and Metabolic Dysfunction," *J. Clin. Invest.* 121, no. 6 (June 2011): 2126–32, doi: 10.1172/JCI58109, Epub June 1, 2011.

11. V. K. Ridaura *et al.*, "Gut Microbiota from Twins Discordant for Obesity Modulate Metabolism in Mice," *Science* 341, no. 6150 (September 6, 2013): 1241214, doi: 10.1126/science.1241214.

12. P. J. Turnbaugh *et al.*, "An Obesity-Associated Gut Microbiome with Increased Capacity for Energy Harvest," *Nature* 444, no. 7122 (December 21, 2006): 1027–31.

13. J. Gerritsen *et al.*, "Intestinal Microbiota in Human Health and Disease: The Impact of Probiotics," *Genes Nutr.* 7, no. 3 (August 2011): 209–40, doi: 10.1007/s12263-011-0229-7, Epub May 27, 2011.

14. Claudia Wallis, "How Gut Bacteria Help Make Us Fat and Thin," *Scientific American* 310, no. 6, June 1, 2014, http://www.scientificamerican.com/article/how-gut-bacteria-help-make-us-fat-and-thin/.

15. "Cleveland Clinic Research Shows Gut Bacteria Byproduct Impacts Heart Failure," Cleveland Clinic, accessed January 12, 2015, http://my.clevelandclinic.org/about-cleveland-clinic/newsroom/releases-videos-newsletters/cleveland-clinic-research-shows-gut-bacteria-byproduct-impacts-heart-failure.

16. C. N. Lumeng and A. R. Saltiel, "Inflammatory Links between Obesity and Metabolic Disease," *J. Clin. Invest.* 121, no. 6 (June 2011): 2111–17, doi: 10.1172/JCI57132, Epub June 1, 2011.

17. H. Yang *et al.*, "Obesity Increases the Production of Proinflammatory Mediators from Adipose Tissue T Cells and Compromises TCR Repertoire Diversity: Implications for Systemic Inflammation and Insulin Resistance," *J. Immunol.* 185, no. 3 (August 1, 2010): 1836–45, doi: 10.4049/jimmunol.1000021, Epub June 25, 2010.

18. W. Jagust *et al.*, "Central Obesity and the Aging Brain," *Arch. Neurol.* 62, no. 10 (October 2005): 1545–48.

19. S. Debette *et al.*, "Visceral Fat Is Associated with Lower Brain Volume in Healthy Middle-Aged Adults," *Ann. Neurol.* 68, no. 2 (August 2010): 136–44, doi: 10.1002/ana.22062.

20. R. Schmidt *et al.*, "Early Inflammation and Dementia: A 25-Year Follow-Up of the Honolulu-Asia Aging Study," *Ann. Neurol.* 52, no. 2 (August 2002): 168–74. See also Joseph Rogers, "High-Sensitivity C-Reactive Protein: An Early Marker of Alzheimer's?," *N. Engl. J. Med. Journal Watch*, October 11, 2002.

21. National Diabetes Statistics Report, 2014, http://www.cdc.gov/diabetes/pubs/statsreport14/national-diabetes-report-web.pdf

22. A.V. Hartstra *et al.*, "Insights into the Role of the Microbiome in Obesity and Type 2 Diabetes," *Diabetes Care* 38, no. 1 (January 2015): 159–165. For a list of publications by Dr. M. Nieuwdorp, go to: https://www.amc.nl/web/Research/Who-is-Who-in-Research/Who-is-Who-in-Research.htm?p=1597&v=publications. Also see R. S. Kootte *et al.*, "The Therapeutic Potential of Manipulating Gut Microbiota in Obesity and Type 2 Diabetes Mellitus," *Diabetes Obes. Metab.* 14, no. 2 (February 2012): 112–20, doi: 10.1111/j.1463-1326.2011.01483.x, Epub November 22, 2011.

23. Turnbaugh *et al.*, "An Obesity-Associated Gut Microbiome."

24. V. K. Ridaura *et al.*, "Gut Microbiota from Twins Discordant for Obesity Modulate Metabolism in Mice."

25. Wallis, "How Gut Bacteria Help Make Us Fat and Thin."

26. T. Poutahidis *et al.*, "Microbial Reprogramming Inhibits Western Diet-Associated Obesity," *PLoS One* 8, no. 7 (July 10, 2013), e68596, doi: 10.1371/journal.pone.0068596.

27. G. A. Bray *et al.*, "Consumption of High-Fructose Corn Syrup in Beverages May Play a Role in the Epidemic of Obesity," *Am. J. Clin. Nutr.* 79, no. 4 (April 2004): 537–43.

28. A. Abbott, "Sugar Substitutes Linked to Obesity," *Nature* 513, no. 7518 (September 18, 2014): 290, doi: 10.1038/513290a.

29. K. K. Ryan *et al.*, "FXR Is a Molecular Target for the Effects of Vertical Sleeve Gastrectomy," *Nature* 509, no. 7499 (May 8, 2014): 183–88, doi: 10.1038/nature13135, Epub March 26, 2014.

30. S. F. Clarke *et al.*, "Exercise and Associated Dietary Extremes Impact on Gut Microbial Diversity," *Gut* 63, no. 12 (December 2014): 1913–20, doi: 10.1136/gutjnl-2013-306541, Epub June 9, 2014.

31. M. C. Arrieta *et al.*, "The Intestinal Microbiome in Early Life: Health and Disease," *Front. Immunol.* 5 (September 5, 2014): 427, doi: 10.3389/fimmu.2014.00427, eCollection 2014.

32. "Early Antibiotic Exposure Leads to Lifelong Metabolic Disturbance in Mice," News Release, NUY Langone Medical Center, August 14, 2014, http://communications

.med.nyu.edu/media-relations/news/early-antibiotic-exposure-leads-lifelong-meta bolic-disturbances-mice. See also L. M. Cox *et al.*, "Altering the Intestinal Micro-biota during a Critical Developmental Window Has Lasting Metabolic Conse-quences," *Cell* 158, no. 4 (August 14, 2014): 705–21, doi: 10.1016/j.cell.2014.05.052.

33. Wallis, "How Gut Bacteria Help Make Us Fat and Thin."
34. Blaser Lab Group, "Lab Overview," accessed January 15, 2015, http://www.med .nyu.edu/medicine/labs/blaserlab/.

Chapter 5: Autism and the Gut

1. Melissa Pandika, "Autism's Gut-Brain Connection," *National Geographic*, Novem-ber 14, 2014, http://news.nationalgeographic.com/news/2014/11/141114-autism-gut -brain-probiotic-research-biology-medicine-bacteria/.
2. "Autism Spectrum Disorder," Centers for Disease Control and Prevention, January 2, 2015, accessed January 12, 2015, http://www.cdc.gov/ncbddd/autism/index.html.
3. Autism Speaks. "Largest-Ever Autism Genome Study Finds Most Siblings Have Different Autism-Risk Genes," *ScienceDaily*, January 26, 2015, www.sciencedaily .com/releases/2015/01/150126124604.htm.
4. Stephen W. Scherer, *et al.* "Whole-genome Sequencing of Quartet Families with Autism Spectrum Disorder," *Nature Medicine*, 2015; doi: 10.1038/nm.3792
5. The chart on page 119, "Autism Spectrum Disorder — Incidence Rates," is based on data from the CDC and National Institutes of Health. It was created by Joanne Marcinek and can be found at http://joannemarcinek.com/autism-spectrum-disorder -incidence-rates/ (accessed January 15, 2015).
6. F. Godiee *et al.*, "Wakefield's Article Linking MMR Vaccine and Autism Was Fraudulent," *BMJ* 342 (January 5, 2011): c7452, doi: 10.1136/bmj.c7452.
7. Melinda Wenner Moyer, "Gut Bacteria May Play a Role in Autism," *Scientific American Mind* 25, no. 5, August 14, 2014, http://www.scientificamerican.com/ article/gut-bacteria-may-play-a-role-in-autism/.
8. H. M. Parracho *et al.*, "Differences between the Gut Microflora of Children with Autistic Spectrum Disorders and That of Healthy Children," *J. Med. Microbiol.* 54, pt. 10 (October 2005): 987–91.
9. Sarah Deweerdt, "New Gene Studies Suggest There Are Hundreds of Kinds of Autism," *Wired*, November 25, 2014, http://www.wired.com/2014/11/autism -genetics/.
10. "Scientists Implicate More Than 100 Genes in Causing Autism," NPR, October 29, 2014, http://www.npr.org/blogs/health/2014/10/29/359818102/scientists-implicate -more-than-100-genes-in-causing-autism.
11. P. Gorrindo *et al.*, "Gastrointestinal Dysfunction in Autism: Parental Report, Clin-ical Evaluation, and Associated Factors," *Autism Res.* 5, no. 2 (April 2012): 101–8, doi: 10.1002/aur.237.

12. L. de Magistris *et al.*, "Alterations of the Intestinal Barrier in Patients with Autism Spectrum Disorders and in Their First-Degree Relatives," *J. Pediatr. Gastroenterol. Nutr.* 51, no. 4 (October 2010): 418–24, doi: 10.1097/MPG.0b013e3181dcc4a5.

13. E. Emanuele *et al.*, "Low-Grade Endotoxemia in Patients with Severe Autism," *Neurosci. Lett.* 471, no. 3 (March 8, 2010): 162–65, doi: 10.1016/j.neulet.2010.01.033, Epub January 25, 2010. The image on page 128 is based on data from this study.

14. J. F. White, "Intestinal Pathophysiology in Autism," *Exp. Biol. Med.* (Maywood) 228, no. 6 (June 2003): 639–49.

15. J. G. Mulle *et al.*, "The Gut Microbiome: A New Frontier in Autism Research," *Curr. Psychiatry Rep.* 15, no. 2 (February 2013): 337, doi: 10.1007/s11920-012-0337-0.

16. S. M. Finegold *et al.*, "Gastrointestinal Microflora Studies in Late-Onset Autism," *Clin. Infect. Dis.* 35, Suppl. 1 (September 1, 2002): S6–S16.

17. Parracho *et al.*, "Differences between the Gut Microflora."

18. R. H. Sandler *et al.*, "Short-Term Benefit from Oral Vancomycin Treatment of Regressive-Onset Autism," *J. Child Neurol.* 15, no. 7 (July 2000): 429–35.

19. Sydney M. Finegold, "Studies on Bacteriology of Autism," accessed January 29, 2015, http://bacteriaandautism.com/.

20. Sandler *et al.*, "Short-Term Benefit from Oral Vancomycin Treatment."

21. Finegold, "Studies on Bacteriology of Autism."

22. Finegold *et al.*, "Gastrointestinal Microflora Studies in Late-Onset Autism."

23. Derrick MacFabe, Western Social Science, The Kilee Patchell-Evans Autism Research Group, accessed January 29, 2015, http://www.psychology.uwo.ca/autism/.

24. D. F. MacFabe, "Short-Chain Fatty Acid Fermentation Products of the Gut Microbiome: Implications in Autism Spectrum Disorders," *Microb. Ecol. Health Dis.* 23 (August 24, 2012), doi: 10.3402/mehd.v23i0.19260, eCollection 2012.

25. S. J. James *et al.*, "Cellular and Mitochondrial Glutathione Redox Imbalance in Lymphoblastoid Cells Derived from Children with Autism," *FASEB J.* 23, no. 8 (August 2009): 2374–83, doi: 10.1096/fj.08-128926, Epub March 23, 2009.

26. A. M. Aldbass *et al.*, "Protective and Therapeutic Potency of N-Acetyl-Cysteine on Propionic Acid-Induced Biochemical Autistic Features in Rats," *J. Neuroinflamm.* 10 (March 27, 2013): 42, doi: 10.1186/1742-2094-10-42.

27. A. Y. Hardan *et al.*, "A Randomized Controlled Pilot Trial of Oral N-Acetylcysteine in Children with Autism," *Biol. Psychiatry* 71, no 11 (June 1, 2012): 956–61, doi: 10.1016/j.biopsych.2012.01.014, Epub February 18, 2012.

28. E. Y. Hsiao *et al.*, "Microbiota Modulate Behavioral and Physiological Abnormalities Associated with Neurodevelopmental Disorders," *Cell* 155, no. 7 (December 19, 2013): 1451–63, doi: 10.1016/j.cell.2013.11.024, Epub December 5, 2013. See also E. Y. Hsiao *et al.*, "Maternal Immune Activation Yields Offspring Displaying Mouse Versions of the Three Core Symptoms of Autism," *Brain Behav. Immun.* 26, no. 4 (May 2012): 607–16, doi: 10.1016/j.bbi.2012.01.011, Epub January 30, 2012.

29. R. E. Frye and D. A. Rossignol, "Mitochondrial Dysfunction Can Connect the Diverse Medical Symptoms Associated with Autism Spectrum Disorders," *Pediatr. Res.* 69, no. 5, pt. 2 (May 2011): 41R–7R, doi: 10.1203/PDR.0b013e318212f16b.

30. P. F. Chinnery, "Mitochondrial Disorders Overview," in *GeneReviews* [Internet], edited by R. A. Pagon *et al.* (Seattle: University of Washington, 1993–2015).

31. C. Giulivi *et al.*, "Mitochondrial Dysfunction in Autism," *JAMA* 304, no. 21 (December 1, 2010): 2389–96, doi: 10.1001/jama.2010.1706.

32. University of California—Davis Health System, "Children with Autism Have Mitochondrial Dysfunction, Study Finds," *ScienceDaily*, accessed January 12, 2015, http://www.sciencedaily.com/releases/2010/11/101130161521.htm .

Chapter 6: Punched in the Gut

1. K. Brown *et al.*, "Diet-Induced Dysbiosis of the Intestinal Microbiota and the Effects on Immunity and Disease," *Nutrients* 4, no. 8 (August 2012): 1095–119, Epub August 21, 2012.

2. J. Suez *et al.*, "Artificial Sweeteners Induce Glucose Intolerance by Altering the Gut Microbiota," *Nature* 514, no. 7521 (October 9, 2014): 181–86, doi: 10.1038/nature13793, Epub September 17, 2014.

3. G. Fagherazzi *et al.*, "Consumption of Artificially and Sugar-Sweetened Beverages and Incident Type 2 Diabetes in the Etude Epidemiologique aupres des Femmes de la Mutuelle Generale de l'Education Nationale-European Prospective Investigation into Cancer and Nutrition Cohort," *Am. J. Clin. Nutr.* 97, no. 3 (March 2013): 517–23, doi: 10.3945/ajcn.112.050997, Epub January 30, 2013. The image on page 147 is based on data from this study.

4. K. Kavanagh *et al.*, "Dietary Fructose Induces Endotoxemia and Hepatic Injury in Calorically Controlled Primates," *Am. J. Clin. Nutr.* 98, no. 2 (August 2013): 349–57, doi: 10.3945/ajcn.112.057331.

5. S. Drago *et al.*, "Gliadin, Zonulin and Gut Permeability: Effects on Celiac and Non-celiac Intestinal Mucosa and Intestinal Cell Lines," *Scand. J. Gastroenterol.* 41, no. 4 (April 2006): 408–19.

6. A. Alaedini *et al.*, "Immune Cross-Reactivity in Celiac Disease: Anti-gliadin Antibodies Bind to Neuronal Synapsin I," *J. Immunol.* 178, no. 10 (May 15, 2007): 6590–95.

7. J. Visser *et al.*, "Tight Junctions, Intestinal Permeability, and Autoimmunity: Celiac Disease and Type 1 Diabetes Paradigms," *Ann. N. Y. Acad. Sci.* 1165 (May 2009): 195–205, doi: 10.1111/j.1749-6632.2009.04037.x.

8. A. Fasano, "Zonulin and Its Regulation of Intestinal Barrier Function: The Biological Door to Inflammation, Autoimmunity, and Cancer," *Physiol. Rev.* 91, no. 1 (January 2011): 151–75, doi: 10.1152/physrev.00003.2008.

9. M. M. Leonard and B. Vasagar, "US Perspective on Gluten-Related Diseases," *Clin. Exp. Gastroenterol.* 7 (January 24, 2014): 25–37, doi: 10.2147/CEG.S54567, eCollection 2014.

10. Brown *et al.*, "Diet-Induced Dysbiosis of the Intestinal Microbiota."

11. E. V. Marietta *et al.*, "Low Incidence of Spontaneous Type 1 Diabetes in Non-obese Diabetic Mice Raised on Gluten-Free Diets Is Associated with Changes in the Intestinal Microbiome," *PLoS One* 8, no. 11 (November 2013): e78687, doi: 10.1371/journal.pone.0078687, eCollection 2013.

12. D. P. Funda *et al.*, "Prevention or Early Cure of Type 1 Diabetes by Intranasal Administration of Gliadin in NOD Mice," *PLoS One* 9, no. 4 (April 11, 2014): e94530, doi: 10.1371/journal.pone.0094530, eCollection 2014.

13. K. Vandepoele and Y. Van de Peer, "Exploring the Plant Transcriptome through Phylogenetic Profiling," *Plant Physiol.* 137, no. 1 (January 2005): 31–42.

Chapter 7: Bust a Gut

1. Centers for Disease Control and Prevention, "Antibiotic Resistance Threats in the United States, 2013," accessible at http://www.cdc.gov/drugresistance/threat-report -2013/pdf/ar-threats-2013-508.pdf (accessed February 4, 2015).

2. "WHO's First Global Report on Antibiotic Resistance Reveals Serious, Worldwide Threat to Public Health," WHO, accessed January 12, 2015, http://www.who.int/ mediacentre/news/releases/2014/amr-report/en/.

3. "Penicillin," Alexander Fleming's Nobel Lecture, December 11, 1945, http://www .nobelprize.org/nobel_prizes/medicine/laureates/1945/fleming-lecture.pdf.

4. "Antibiotic/Antimicrobial Resistance," Centers for Disease Control and Prevention, accessed January 29, 2015, http://www.cdc.gov/drugresistance/.

5. F. Francois *et al.*, "The Effect of *H. pylori* Eradication on Meal-Associated Changes in Plasma Ghrelin and Leptin," *BMC Gastroenterol.* 11 (April 14, 2011): 37, doi: 10.1186/1471-230X-11-37.

6. The image on page 160 is adapted from James Byrne, *Disease Prone* blog on ScientificAmerican.com, http://blogs.scientificamerican.com/disease-prone/files/ 2011/11/ABx-use-graph.png.

7. David Kessler, "Antibiotics and Meat We Eat," *New York Times*, March 27, 2013, Opinion Page, A27, http://www.nytimes.com/2013/03/28/opinion/antibiotics-and -the-meat-we-eat.html.

8. Ibid.

9. C. J. Hildreth *et al.*, "JAMA Patient Page. Inappropriate Use of Antibiotics," *JAMA* 302, no. 7 (August 19, 2009): 816, doi: 10.1001/jama.302.7.816.

10. C. M. Velicer *et al.*, "Antibiotic Use in Relation to the Risk of Breast Cancer," *JAMA* 291, no. 7 (February 18, 2004): 827–35. The image on page 162 is based on data from this study.

11. R. F. Schwabe and C. Jobin, "The Microbiome and Cancer," *Nat. Rev. Cancer* 13, no. 11 (November 2013): 800–812, doi: 10.1038/nrc3610, Epub October 17, 2013.

12. U.S. Food and Drug Administration, "FDA Drug Safety Communication: Azithromycin (Zithromax or Zmax) and the Risk of Potentially Fatal Heart Rhythms," accessed January 12, 2015, http://www.fda.gov/Drugs/DrugSafety/ucm341822.htm.

13. Michael O'Riordan, "Cardiac Risks with Antibiotics Azithromycin, Levofloxacin Supported by VA Data," Medscape, March 10, 2014, http://www.medscape.com/viewarticle/821697.

14. T. R. Coker *et al.*, "Diagnosis, Microbial Epidemiology, and Antibiotic Treatment of Acute Otitis Media in Children: A Systematic Review," *JAMA* 304, no. 19 (November 17, 2010): 2161–69, doi: 10.1001/jama.2010.1651.

15. E. F. Berbari *et al.*, "Dental Procedures as Risk Factors for Prosthetic Hip or Knee Infection: A Hospital-Based Prospective Case-Control Study," *Clin. Infect. Dis.* 50, no. 1 (January 1, 2010): 8–16, doi: 10.1086/648676.

16. Kathleen Doheny, "Birth Control Pills, HRT Tied to Digestive Ills," HealthDay, May 21, 2012, http://consumer.healthday.com/women-s-health-information-34/birth-control-news-62/birth-control-pills-hrt-tied-to-digestive-ills-664939.html.

17. H. Khalili *et al.*, "Oral Contraceptives, Reproductive Factors and Risk of Inflammatory Bowel Disease," *Gut* 62, no. 8 (August 2013): 1153–59, doi: 10.1136/gutjnl-2012-302362, Epub May 22, 2012.

18. Kelly Brogan, "Holistic Women's Health Psychiatry," accessed January 29, 2015, http://www.kellybroganmd.com.

19. K. Andersen *et al.*, "Do Nonsteroidal Anti-inflammatory Drugs Decrease the Risk for Alzheimer's Disease? The Rotterdam Study," *Neurology* 45, no. 8 (August 1995): 1441–45.

20. J. M. Natividad *et al.*, "Host Responses to Intestinal Microbial Antigens in Gluten-Sensitive Mice," *PLoS One* 4, no. 7 (July 31, 2009): e6472, doi: 10.1371/journal.pone.0006472.

21. The Environmental Working Group, "Toxic Chemicals Found in Minority Cord Blood," News Release, December 2, 2009; accessible at http://www.ewg.org/news/news-releases/2009/12/02/toxic-chemicals-found-minority-cord-blood (accessed February 4, 2015).

22. The Environmental Protection Agency: http://www.epa.gov.

23. The Environmental Working Group: http://www.ewg.org.

24. H. S. Lee *et al.*, "Associations among Organochlorine Pesticides, Methanobacteriales, and Obesity in Korean Women," *PLoS One* 6, no. 11 (2011): e27773, doi: 10.1371/journal.pone.0027773, Epub November 17, 2011.

25. *Life* magazine, volume 20, no.10a, Fall 1997.

26. "Global Water Soluble Fertilizers Market, by Types (Nitrogenous, Phosphatic, Potassic, Micronutrients), Applications (Fertigation, Foliar Application), Crop Types (Field, Horticultural, Turf & Ornamentals) & Geography — Trends & Forecasts to

2017," PR Newswire, March 6, 2013, http://www.prnewswire.com/news-releases/global -water-soluble-fertilizers-market-by-types-nitrogenous-phosphatic-potassic-micro nutrients-applications-fertigation-foliar-application-crop-types-field-horticultural-turf --ornamentals--geography---trends--f-195525101.html (accessed February 4, 2015).

27. S. Seneff and A. Samsel, "Glyphosate, Pathways to Modern Diseases II: Celiac Sprue and Gluten Intolerance," *Interdiscip. Toxicol.* 6, no. 4 (December 2013): 159–84, doi: 10.2478/intox-2013-0026. The image on page 174 is extracted from published paper (Copyright © 2013 SETOX & IEPT, SASc.), which is an Open Access article distributed under the terms of the Creative Commons Attribution License (http://creativecommons.org/licenses/by/2.0).

28. Ibid.

29. "Where GMOs Hide in Your Food," *Consumer Reports*, October 2014, http://www .ConsumerReports.org/cro/gmo1014.

Chapter 8: Feeding Your Microbiome

1. "Ilya Mechnikov — Biographical," Nobelprize.org, accessed January 29, 2015, http://www.nobelprize.org/nobel_prizes/medicine/laureates/1908/mechnikov-bio .html.

2. G. W. Tannock, "A Special Fondness for Lactobacilli," *Appl. Environ. Microbiol.* 70, no. 6 (June 2004): 3189–94.

3. P. K. Elias *et al.*, "Serum Cholesterol and Cognitive Performance in the Framingham Heart Study," *Psychosom. Med.* 67, no. 1 (January–February 2005): 24–30.

4. M. Mulder *et al.*, "Reduced Levels of Cholesterol, Phospholipids, and Fatty Acids in Cerebrospinal Fluid of Alzheimer Disease Patients Are Not Related to Apolipoprotein E4," *Alzheimer Dis. Assoc. Disord.* 12, no. 3 (September 1998): 198–203.

5. C. B. Ebbeling *et al.*, "Effects of Dietary Composition on Energy Expenditure during Weight-Loss Maintenance," *JAMA* 307, no. 24 (June 27, 2012): 2627–34, doi: 10.1001/jama.2012.6607.

6. S. Moco, F. P. Martin, and S. Rezzi, "Metabolomics View on Gut Microbiome Modulation by Polyphenol-Rich Foods," *J. Proteome Res.* 11, no. 10 (October 5, 2012): 4781–90, doi: 10.1021/pr300581s, Epub September 6, 2012.

7. F. Cardona *et al.*, "Benefits of Polyphenols on Gut Microbiota and Implications in Human Health," *J. Nutr. Biochem.* 24, no. 8 (August 2013): 1415–22, doi: 10.1016/j .jnutbio.2013.05.001.

8. D. C. Vodnar and C. Socaciu, "Green Tea Increases the Survival Yield of Bifidobacteria in Simulated Gastrointestinal Environment and during Refrigerated Conditions," *Chem. Cent. J.* 6, no. 1 (June 22, 2012): 61, doi: 10.1186/1752-153X-6-61.

9. G. Desideri *et al.*, "Benefits in Cognitive Function, Blood Pressure, and Insulin Resistance through Cocoa Flavanol Consumption in Elderly Subjects with Mild Cognitive Impairment: The Cocoa, Cognition, and Aging (CoCoA) Study,"

Hypertension 60, no. 3 (September 2012): 794–801, doi: 10.1161/HYPERTENSIO NAHA.112.193060, Epub August 14, 2012.

10. S. T. Francis *et al.*, "The Effect of Flavanol-Rich Cocoa on the fMRI Response to a Cognitive Task in Healthy Young People," *J. Cardiovasc. Pharmacol.* 47, Suppl. 2 (2006): S215–20.

11. "Drinking Cocoa Boosts Cognition and Blood Flow in the Brain," *Tufts University Health & Nutrition Letter*, November 2013, http://www.nutritionletter.tufts.edu/ issues/9_11/current-articles/Drinking-Cocoa-Boosts-Cognition-and-Blood-Flow -in-the-Brain_1270-1.html.

12. M. Clemente-Postigo *et al.*, "Effect of Acute and Chronic Red Wine Consumption on Lipopolysaccharide Concentrations," *Am. J. Clin. Nutr.* 97, no. 5 (May 2013): 1053–61, doi: 10.3945/ajcn.112.051128, Epub April 10, 2013.

13. J. Slavin, "Fiber and Prebiotics: Mechanisms and Health Benefits," *Nutrients* 5, no. 4 (April 22, 2013): 1417–35, doi: 10.3390/nu5041417.

14. Ibid.

15. R. J. Colman *et al.*, "Caloric Restriction Delays Disease Onset and Mortality in Rhesus Monkeys," *Science* 325, no. 5937 (July 10, 2009): 201–4, doi: 10.1126/ science.1173635.

16. Jessica Firger, "Calorie-Restricted Diet May Help Keep the Mind Sharp," CBS News, November 18, 2014, http://www.cbsnews.com/news/calorie-restricted-diet -may-slow-aging-cognitive-mental-decline/.

17. C. Zhang *et al.*, "Structural Modulation of Gut Microbiota in Life-Long Calorie -Restricted Mice," *Nat. Commun.* 4 (2013): 2163, doi: 10.1038/ncomms3163.

Chapter 9: Go Pro

1. P. Ducrotte, P. Sawant, and V. Jayanthi, "Clinical Trial: *Lactobacillus plantarum* 299v (DSM 9843) Improves Symptoms of Irritable Bowel Syndrome," *World J. Gastroenterol.* 18, no. 30 (August 14, 2012): 4012–18, doi: 10.3748/wjg.v18.i30.4012.

2. Adlam, Katie, "*Lactobacillus plantarum* and Its Biological Implications," Microbe-Wiki, Kenyon College, https://microbewiki.kenyon.edu/index.php/Lactobacillus _plantarum_and_its_biological_implications.

3. "*Lactobacillus acidophilus*," University of Maryland Medical Center, Medical Reference Guide, http://umm.edu/health/medical/altmed/supplement/lactobacillus -acidophilus.

4. "*Lactobacillus brevis*," MicrobeWiki, Kenyon College, https://microbewiki.kenyon .edu/index.php/Lactobacillus_brevis.

5. E. O'Sullivan *et al.*, "BDNF Expression in the Hippocampus of Maternally Separated Rats: Does *Bifidobacterium breve* 6330 Alter BDNF Levels?," *Benef. Microbes* 2, no. 3 (September 2011): 199–207, doi: 10.3920/BM2011.0015.

6. "Bifidobacteria," Medline Plus, http://www.nlm.nih.gov/medlineplus/druginfo/natural/891.html.

7. D. Guyonnet *et al.*, "Fermented Milk Containing *Bifidobacterium lactis* DN-173 010 Improved Self-Reported Digestive Comfort amongst a General Population of Adults: A Randomized, Open-Label, Controlled, Pilot Study," *J. Dig. Dis.* 10, no. 1 (February 2009): 61–70, doi: 10.1111/j.1751-2980.2008.00366.x.

8. G. Rizzardini *et al.*, "Evaluation of the Immune Benefits of Two Probiotic Strains *Bifidobacterium animalis ssp. lactis*, BB-12® and *Lactobacillus paracasei ssp. paracasei, L. casei 431®* in an Influenza Vaccination Model: A Randomised, Double-Blind, Placebo-Controlled Study," *Br. J. Nutr.* 107, no. 6 (March 2012): 876–84, doi: 10.1017/S000711451100420X, Epub September 7, 2011.

9. "*Bifidobacterium longum*," MicrobeWiki, Kenyon College, https://microbewiki.kenyon.edu/index.php/Bifidobacterium_longum.

10. F. Savino *et al.*, "*Lactobacillus reuteri* (American Type Culture Collection Strain 55730) versus Simethicone in the Treatment of Infantile Colic: A Prospective Randomized Study," *Pediatrics* 119, no. 1 (January 2007): e124–30.

11. H. Szymanski *et al.*, "Treatment of Acute Infectious Diarrhoea in Infants and Children with a Mixture of Three *Lactobacillus rhamnosus* Strains—a Randomized, Double-Blind, Placebo-Controlled Trial," *Aliment. Pharmacol. Ther.* 23, no. 2 (January 2006): 247–53.

12. M. Kalliomaki *et al.*, "Probiotics in Primary Prevention of Atopic Disease: A Randomised Placebo-Controlled Trial," *Lancet* 375, no. 9262 (April 7, 2001): 1076–69.

13. J. H. Ooi *et al.*, "Vitamin D Regulates the Gut Microbiome and Protects Mice from Dextran Sodium Sulfate-Induced Colitis," *J. Nutr.* 143, no. 10 (October 2013): 1679–86, doi: 10.3945/jn.113.180794, Epub August 21, 2013.

Epilogue: What the Future Holds

1. David Agus, *The End of Illness* (New York: Free Press, 2009).

2. I. Youngster *et al.*, "Oral, Capsulized, Frozen Fecal Microbiota Transplantation for Relapsing *Clostridium difficile* Infection," *JAMA* 312, no. 17 (November 5, 2014): 1772–78, doi: 10.1001/jama.2014.13875.

3. Emily Hollister, "Fresh Infusions: The Science behind Fecal Transplants," Baylor College of Medicine, http://www.asmbranches.org/brcano/meetings/2014SprPpts/4.3Hollister_NCASM_2014.pdf.

4. Els van Nood *et al.*, "Fecal Microbiota Transplantation," *Curr. Opin. Gastroenterol.* 30, no. 1 (2014): 34–39.

5. "What Is FMT?," The Fecal Transplant Foundation, http://thefecaltransplant foundation.org/what-is-fecal-transplant/.

6. T. J. Borody *et al.*, "Fecal Microbiota Transplantation: Indications, Methods, Evidence, and Future Directions," *Curr. Gastroenterol. Rep.* 15, no. 8 (August 2013): 337, doi: 10.1007/s11894-013-0337-1.

7. T. J. Borody *et al.*, "Therapeutic Faecal Microbiota Transplantation: Current Status and Future Developments," *Curr. Opin. Gastroenterol.* 30, no. 1 (January 2014): 97–105, doi: 10.1097/MOG.0000000000000027.

8. T. J. Borody *et al.*, Case Studies #941, 942, *Am. J. Gastroenterol.* 106, Suppl. 2 (October 2011): S352.

9. Kerry Brewster, "Doctor Tom Borody Claims Faecal Transplants Curing Incurable Diseases like Crohn's," ABC News Australia, March 2014, http://www.abc.net.au/news/2014-03-18/sydney-doctor-claims-poo-transplants-curing-diseases/5329836.

10. "For Medical Professionals: Quick, Inexpensive and a 90 Percent Cure Rate," accessed January 13, 2015, http://www.mayoclinic.org/medical-professionals/clinical-updates/digestive-diseases/quick-inexpensive-90-percent-cure-rate.

11. Ferris Jabr, "For the Good of the Gut: Can Parasitic Worms Treat Autoimmune Diseases?," *Scientific American*, December 1, 2010, http://www.scientificamerican.com/article/helminthic-therapy-mucus/

12. M. J. Broadhurst *et al.*, "IL-22+ CD4+ T Cells Are Associated with Therapeutic *Trichuris trichiura* Infection in an Ulcerative Colitis Patient," *Sci. Transl. Med.* 2, no. 60 (December 1, 2010): 60ra88, doi: 10.1126/scitranslmed.3001500.

13. R. W. Summers *et al.*, "*Trichuris suis* Therapy for Active Ulcerative Colitis: A Randomized Controlled Trial," *Gastroenterology* 128, no. 4 (April 2005): 825–32.

14. Katherine Harmon Courage, "Parasitic Worm Eggs Ease Intestinal Ills by Changing Gut Macrobiota," *Scientific American Blogs*, November 15, 2012, http://blogs.scientificamerican.com/observations/2012/11/15/parasitic-worm-eggs-ease-intestinal-ills-by-changing-gut-macrobiota/.

15. S. Reardon, "Gut-Brain Link Grabs Neuroscientists," *Nature* 515 (November 13, 2014): 175–77, doi: 10.1038/515175a.

Index

About the Author

DAVID PERLMUTTER, MD, is a board-certified neurologist and Fellow of the American College of Nutrition. He is president of the Perlmutter Health Center in Naples, Florida, and the cofounder and president of the Perlmutter Brain Foundation. Dr. Perlmutter serves as a volunteer associate professor at the University of Miami School of Medicine. Dr. Perlmutter has been interviewed on many nationally syndicated radio and television programs including *20/20*, *Larry King Live*, *CNN*, *Fox News*, *Fox and Friends*, *The Today Show*, *Oprah*, *Dr. Oz*, and *The CBS Early Show* and serves as medical advisor to the Dr. Oz Show. In 2002 Dr. Perlmutter was the recipient of the Linus Pauling Award for his innovative approaches to neurological disorders and in addition was awarded the Denham Harmon Award for his pioneering work in the application of free radical science to clinical medicine. He is the recipient of the 2006 National Nutritional Foods Association Clinician of the Year Award and was awarded the 2010 Humanitarian of the Year award from the American College of Nutrition. He has contributed extensively to the world medical literature with publications appearing in *The Journal of Neurosurgery*, *The Southern Medical Journal*, *Journal of Applied Nutrition*, and *Archives of Neurology*. He is the author of seven books including the #1 *New York Times* bestseller *Grain Brain*.